RENAL DIET COOKBOOK FOR BEGINNERS

A Complete Guide to Thriving with Kidney Disease Through a Collection of Healthy & Tasty Low Sodium, Potassium, and Phosphorus Recipes for Enhanced Well-Being

Elisa Cooper

HERE IS YOUR FREE GIFT!

SCAN HERE TO DOWNLOAD IT ☝

or:

CLICK HERE TO DOWNLOAD IT 👇

https://elisacooper.aweb.page/p/e992a266-3c48-4cbb-99bd-d5400bc5e0b3

🍽 **1. DINING OUT AND SPECIAL OCCASIONS BEST GUIDE**

🍽 **2. BEST RENAL FLAVORS FROM THE WORLD**

Table of Contents

Introduction

The kidneys are essential organs in the human body, responsible for filtering waste and extra fluids from the blood, regulating electrolytes, and maintaining overall fluid balance. A well-functioning pair of kidneys is vital for our overall health and well-being. Unfortunately, many individuals suffer from kidney diseases or disorders that impair their kidney function. For these individuals, a renal diet plays a crucial role in managing and improving kidney health.

What is a Renal Diet?

A renal diet, also known as a kidney diet, is a specialized eating plan tailored to the unique dietary needs of individuals with kidney disease or impaired kidney function. The primary goal of a renal diet is to reduce the burden on the kidneys and maintain optimal health by managing specific aspects of nutrient intake. Let's delve deeper into the key components of a renal diet.

Nutrient Control

The cornerstone of a renal diet is careful control of nutrients, including protein, sodium, potassium, and phosphorus. The kidneys play a central role in regulating these substances in the body. When kidney function is impaired, these elements can accumulate to dangerous levels, leading to various complications.

- **Protein Control:** Protein is an essential part of a healthy diet, but for individuals with kidney disease, excessive protein intake can strain the kidneys. A renal diet typically limits the amount of protein consumed, particularly high-quality protein sources such as red meat, poultry, and fish. Instead, it encourages the consumption of high biological value (HBV) proteins like egg whites and plant-based sources, as they produce fewer waste products that the kidneys need to filter.
- **Sodium Control:** Sodium, frequently present in table salt and processed food items, may lead to elevated blood pressure and the retention of extra fluids. A renal diet restricts sodium intake to help manage blood pressure and prevent the retention of extra fluids. This is essential for individuals with kidney disease, as it reduces the workload on their already compromised kidneys.
- **Potassium Control:** Potassium is essential for nerve and muscle function, but elevated levels can be harmful to those with kidney disease. A renal diet helps manage potassium intake, often by limiting high-potassium foods such as bananas, oranges, and potatoes. Proper potassium control helps prevent heart and muscle problems that can arise from extra potassium.
- **Phosphorus Control:** Phosphorus is found in many foods, especially in protein-rich sources, and is typically taken out from the body through the kidneys. In kidney disease, impaired filtration can lead to phosphorus buildup, which can weaken bones and damage blood vessels. A renal diet addresses this by limiting phosphorus intake and prescribing phosphorus binders to reduce absorption.

Fluid Management

The kidneys are responsible for maintaining the body's fluid balance. In kidney disease, this function is often compromised, leading to fluid retention and swelling. A renal diet helps individuals manage their fluid intake, preventing excessive fluid buildup and associated complications.

Calorie Control
Ensuring an optimal weight is essential in the management of kidney disease. Consuming excessive calories can result in weight gain, while insufficient calorie intake may lead to muscle loss and weakness. A renal diet aims to provide the right amount of calories for each individual, considering factors like age, activity level, and overall health.

Micronutrient Optimization
In addition to controlling macronutrients like protein, sodium, potassium, and phosphorus, a renal diet focuses on optimizing micronutrient intake. This includes ensuring that individuals with kidney disease receive adequate vitamins and minerals, such as vitamin D, calcium, and iron, which may be compromised by dietary restrictions.

Individualized Meal Plans
It's crucial to emphasize that renal diets are not universally applicable. The dietary guidelines can differ based on the stage and nature of kidney disease, as well as individual factors like age, gender, and overall health. Registered dietitians with expertise in renal nutrition often work closely with patients to develop personalized meal plans that meet their unique needs.

Importance of A Renal Diet for Renal Kidney Health

The importance of following a renal diet for renal kidney health cannot be overstated. Kidney disease, whether acute or chronic, significantly impacts the body's ability to filter waste and maintain proper fluid balance. Consequently, adhering to a renal diet can make a substantial difference in an individual's overall well-being. Let's explore the key reasons why a renal diet is crucial for maintaining renal kidney health.

- **Slowing Disease Progression:** For individuals with chronic kidney disease (CKD), slowing down the progression of the disease is of paramount importance. A renal diet, through its careful control of nutrients, helps reduce the workload on the kidneys. This, in turn, can slow the decline in kidney function and potentially delay the need for dialysis or transplantation.

- **Blood Pressure Management:** High blood pressure is a common complication of kidney disease and can further damage the kidneys. By limiting sodium intake and promoting a heart-healthy diet, a renal diet aids in the management of blood pressure, reducing the risk of cardiovascular events and further kidney damage.

- **Fluid Balance:** Proper fluid balance is essential to avoid fluid retention and swelling, common problems in kidney disease. A renal diet helps individuals manage their fluid intake, preventing these complications and enhancing their overall comfort and quality of life.

- **Electrolyte Control:** The kidneys are responsible for maintaining the body's electrolyte balance, and kidney disease can disrupt this balance. A renal diet, which carefully controls potassium and phosphorus intake, plays a critical role in preventing electrolyte imbalances and their associated complications, such as muscle weakness and heart irregularities.

- **Improved Nutritional Status:** Despite the dietary restrictions, a well-planned renal diet can provide individuals with kidney disease the essential nutrients they need to maintain good health. Nutrient optimization is a fundamental aspect of renal nutrition, ensuring that patients receive the right balance of vitamins and minerals to support their overall well-being.

- **Enhanced Quality of Life:** By addressing the dietary challenges posed by kidney disease, a renal diet can enhance the quality of life for individuals affected by this condition. It reduces symptoms, such as fatigue and edema, and helps individuals regain a sense of control over their health.
- **Prevention of Complications:** Kidney disease can lead to various complications, including anemia, bone disease, and cardiovascular problems. A renal diet, by managing nutrients and fluids, aids in preventing or minimizing these complications, thereby reducing the overall burden on individuals with kidney disease.
- **Individualized Care:** Every person's kidney disease is unique, and their dietary needs may differ based on various factors. A renal diet is tailored to the individual, ensuring that they receive the specific care and support they require.
- **Collaborative Approach:** In addition to diet, managing kidney disease often involves medications, regular monitoring, and lifestyle modifications. A renal diet is just one piece of the puzzle in kidney disease management. A multidisciplinary approach, involving nephrologists, dietitians, nurses, and other healthcare professionals, is essential to provide holistic care and support to individuals with kidney disease.
- **Long-Term Kidney Health:** A renal diet is not a short-term fix but a long-term commitment to kidney health. By consistently following a renal diet, individuals with kidney disease can work toward maintaining their kidney function and preserving their quality of life.

CHAPTER 1: Understanding Kidney Disease

The kidneys are remarkable organs with a crucial role in maintaining overall health and well-being. However, kidney disease can affect their function, leading to various health complications. Here, we will delve into understanding kidney disease, including the most common types and their related stages. We will also explore the essential nutritional principles for kidney health and lifestyle tips to follow in managing kidney disease.

Most Common Types of Kidney Disease (KD) And Related Stages

Kidney disease, also known as renal disease, encompasses a wide range of conditions that can affect the kidneys. Understanding the most common types and their related stages is fundamental for effective management and treatment.

Chronic Kidney Disease (CKD)

Chronic Kidney Disease (CKD) is one of the most prevalent and serious types of kidney disease. It is a progressive condition characterized by the gradual loss of kidney function over time. CKD is typically categorized into 5 stages, with stage 1 being the mildest and stage 5 indicating end-stage renal disease (ESRD).

- **Stage 1 - Kidney Damage with Normal GFR:** In stage 1 CKD, there is evidence of kidney damage (such as proteinuria or abnormal imaging) but normal or near-normal kidney function as measured by the glomerular filtration rate (GFR). The GFR is a measure of how well the kidneys filter waste from the blood.

- **Stage 2 - Mild Decrease in GFR:** Stage 2 CKD involves a mild decrease in GFR (90-89 mL/min). Kidney damage is still present, but there is some loss of function.

- **Stage 3 - Moderate Decrease in GFR:** In stage 3, there is a moderate decrease in GFR (59-30 mL/min). It is further divided into two sub-stages: 3A and 3B, based on the severity of GFR decline.

- **Stage 4 - Severe Decrease in GFR:** Stage 4 CKD signifies a severe decrease in GFR (29-15 mL/min). At this stage, kidney function is significantly impaired, and patients may begin to experience symptoms and complications.

- **Stage 5 - End-Stage Renal Disease (ESRD):** ESRD, often referred to as stage 5 CKD, is the most advanced stage of chronic kidney disease. GFR is below 15 mL/min, and patients with ESRD typically require renal replacement therapy, such as dialysis or kidney transplantation, to maintain life.

Acute Kidney Injury (AKI)

Acute Kidney Injury (AKI) is a sudden and rapid loss of kidney function. It can result from a range of factors, such as severe infections, medication usage, dehydration, or trauma. AKI is classified into three stages based on the extent of kidney damage and changes in serum creatinine levels.

- **Stage 1 - Increase in Serum Creatinine:** In stage 1 AKI, there is a mild increase in serum creatinine, which is a marker of kidney function. This may be accompanied by decreased urine output.

- **Stage 2 - Moderate Increase in Serum Creatinine:** Stage 2 AKI involves a moderate increase in serum creatinine, indicating more substantial kidney damage. Urine output continues to decline.
- **Stage 3 - Severe Increase in Serum Creatinine:** Stage 3 AKI is the most severe form, with a significant increase in serum creatinine and a sharp decrease in urine output. Patients in this stage often require immediate medical intervention.

Polycystic Kidney Disease (PKD)

Polycystic Kidney Disease (PKD) is a genetic disorder that leads to the formation of numerous fluid-filled cysts in the kidneys. Over time, these cysts can enlarge, causing damage to the kidney tissue and affecting kidney function. PKD can progress to advanced stages, ultimately leading to kidney failure.

Diabetic Nephropathy

Diabetic nephropathy is a prevalent complication of diabetes. It manifests when prolonged elevated blood sugar levels cause damage to the tiny blood vessels within the kidneys. This condition advances gradually and poses a heightened risk of developing chronic kidney disease (CKD), particularly in individuals with poorly managed diabetes.

Hypertensive Nephropathy

Hypertensive nephropathy, also known as hypertensive kidney disease, results from prolonged high blood pressure. With the passage of time, uncontrolled hypertension can result in harm to the minute blood vessels within the kidneys, potentially leading to kidney dysfunction and, in certain instances, chronic kidney disease (CKD).

Glomerulonephritis

Glomerulonephritis is characterized by inflammation of the glomeruli, the small filtering units within the kidneys. This inflammation can be instigated by infections, autoimmune disorders, or various other factors. Glomerulonephritis can progress to CKD if not properly managed.

Kidney Stones

Kidney stones are small, hard mineral deposits that can form in the kidneys. While kidney stones themselves are not a type of kidney disease, they can cause acute kidney injury if they obstruct the flow of urine. Recurrent kidney stones may also contribute to chronic kidney disease.

Congenital Kidney Conditions

Some individuals are born with congenital kidney conditions, such as renal agenesis (absence of one or both kidneys), renal dysplasia (abnormal kidney development), or obstructive uropathy (blockage of the urinary tract). These conditions can lead to various kidney-related problems throughout life.

Nutritional Principles for Kidney Health and Lifestyle Tips to Follow

Nutrition and lifestyle hold a pivotal role in both the management and prevention of kidney disease. Sustaining a wholesome diet and adopting a healthy lifestyle can contribute to decelerating the advancement of kidney disease, mitigating complications, and enhancing overall well-being. Here are key nutritional principles and lifestyle tips for kidney health:

1. **Hydration**

Drink Plenty of Water Staying well-hydrated is essential for kidney health. It helps flush toxins & waste products from the body and prevents the formation of kidney stones. Aim to drink enough water to keep your urine light yellow in color, but be mindful not to overhydrate, which can strain the kidneys.

2. **Sodium (Salt) Control**

Excessive sodium intake can lead to high blood pressure and fluid retention, both of which are harmful to the kidneys. To control sodium intake:

- Read food labels and choose low-sodium or sodium-free products.
- Limit the use of table salt in cooking and seasoning.
- Avoid high-sodium processed foods, such as tinned soups and fast food.

3. **Potassium Management**

In kidney disease, the kidneys may struggle to regulate potassium levels. To manage potassium intake:

- Limit high-potassium foods like bananas, oranges, and potatoes.
- Choose lower-potassium alternatives, such as apples or cauliflower.
- Avoid salt substitutes that are high in potassium.

4. **Phosphorus Restriction**

Elevated phosphorus levels can lead to bone problems in kidney disease. To control phosphorus intake:

- Limit high-phosphorus foods, including dairy, nuts, and colas.
- Take prescribed phosphorus binders with meals to reduce absorption.

5. **Protein Moderation**

While protein is essential for health, excessive protein intake can strain the kidneys. For kidney health:

- Work with a dietitian to determine your individual protein needs.
- Choose high-biological-value (HBV) proteins like egg whites and lean meat.
- Balance protein intake with your overall dietary plan.

6. **Exercise and Physical Activity**

Regular exercise can benefit kidney health by improving cardiovascular fitness and reducing the risk of complications like diabetes and hypertension. Aim for almost 150 mins of moderate-intensity exercise per week, as recommended by health authorities.

7. **Weight Management**

Sustaining a healthy weight is of paramount importance for kidney health, as obesity constitutes a risk factor for kidney disease and its associated complications. A well-balanced diet coupled with consistent exercise can be instrumental in effectively managing weight.

8. **Smoking Cessation**

Smoking is a contributing risk factor for kidney disease and can exacerbate its progression. Quitting smoking is a vital step in improving kidney health and overall well-being.

9. **Blood Pressure Control**

Hypertension is a prevalent complication of kidney disease. Follow your healthcare provider's recommendations for monitoring and controlling blood pressure, which may include medications, diet, and lifestyle changes.

10. **Medication Management**

If you have received prescriptions for kidney disease or related conditions like diabetes or hypertension, it's crucial to adhere to the prescribed medication regimen. Regularly schedule follow-up appointments with your healthcare provider to ensure the effective management of your condition.

11. Regular Check-ups

Routine check-ups and monitoring of kidney function are essential for detecting and managing kidney disease early. Regular visits to a nephrologist or healthcare provider can help ensure that any changes in kidney function are promptly addressed.

12. Stress Management

Chronic stress can exert an adverse influence on kidney health. Incorporate stress-reduction techniques like meditation, deep breathing exercises, or relaxation therapies into your routine to enhance your overall well-being.

13. Dietary Guidance from a Registered Dietitian

Work with a registered dietitian who specializes in renal nutrition to develop a personalized dietary plan tailored to your specific needs and preferences. Regular consultations with a dietitian can help you maintain a balanced diet that supports kidney health.

CHAPTER 2: Benefits of A Renal Diet

A renal diet, also known as a kidney diet, is a specialized eating plan tailored to the unique dietary needs of individuals with kidney disease or impaired kidney function. While it may seem restrictive, a renal diet offers a multitude of benefits that are crucial for the overall health and well-being of patients with kidney disease.

Benefits of A Renal Diet for Patients with KD

1. Dietary Guidance

One of the primary benefits of a renal diet is the provision of clear and structured dietary guidance. Individuals with kidney disease often face complex dietary challenges due to their impaired kidney function. A renal diet provides them with a roadmap for making informed food choices that support kidney health and minimize further damage. Here are some key aspects of dietary guidance within a renal diet:

- **Nutrient Control:** A renal diet emphasizes the careful control of nutrients such as protein, sodium, potassium, and phosphorus. By adhering to these dietary restrictions, patients can significantly reduce the workload on their kidneys and prevent complications related to the accumulation of these substances.

- **Personalized Meal Plans:** Each individual's kidney disease is unique, with different stages and dietary requirements. Registered dietitians with expertise in renal nutrition work closely with patients to create personalized meal plans tailored to their specific needs, considering factors like the stage of kidney disease, age, gender, activity level, and overall health.

- **Portion Control:** Portion control is essential in a renal diet to manage calorie intake and prevent overconsumption of nutrients that need to be restricted. Patients learn to measure portions and understand the nutritional content of the foods they eat.

- **Label Reading:** Understanding food labels is crucial for individuals with kidney disease. Renal diet guidance includes teaching patients how to read labels and identify high-sodium, high-potassium, or high-phosphorus foods to make informed choices while grocery shopping.

- **Meal Planning:** A renal diet helps patients plan well-balanced meals that align with their dietary restrictions. This includes the selection of foods from various food groups, portion sizes, and the timing of meals and snacks to maintain stable blood sugar levels.

2. Nutritional Balance

A renal diet places a strong emphasis on maintaining nutritional balance. This is critical for individuals with kidney disease, as their dietary restrictions can increase the risk of malnutrition and nutrient deficiencies. Here are some ways in which a renal diet helps achieve nutritional balance:

- **Protein Optimization:** While a renal diet limits overall protein intake, it ensures that patients receive the appropriate amount of high-quality protein. High-biological-value (HBV) proteins, such as egg whites and lean meat, produce fewer waste products that the kidneys need to filter.

- **Micronutrient Support:** The diet also addresses the optimization of micronutrients, including vitamins and minerals like vitamin D, calcium, and iron. These micronutrients are carefully managed to maintain bone health, blood pressure, and overall well-being.
- **Adequate Caloric Intake:** It's essential that individuals with kidney disease consume enough calories to maintain a healthy weight and energy levels. A renal diet helps them determine the appropriate caloric intake based on factors like age, activity level, and overall health.
- **Phosphorus Control:** Phosphorus restriction is a key element of renal nutrition. Patients are guided in managing phosphorus intake through dietary choices and, when necessary, phosphorus binders to reduce absorption.

3. **Kidney Stress Reduction**

Reducing stress and the workload on the kidneys is one of the central objectives of a renal diet. Kidney stress reduction is crucial for slowing the progression of kidney disease and preserving kidney function. Here's how a renal diet achieves this goal:

- **Protein Moderation:** Excessive protein intake can strain the kidneys by producing waste products that need to be filtered. By controlling protein intake and selecting high-quality protein sources, a renal diet eases the burden on the kidneys, reducing their stress.
- **Sodium (Salt) Control:** Sodium is a major factor contributing to high blood pressure and fluid retention. A renal diet helps individuals manage their sodium intake, reducing the stress on the kidneys and preventing hypertension-related complications.
- **Fluid Management:** The kidneys are responsible for regulating the body's fluid balance. In kidney disease, this function is often compromised, leading to fluid retention and swelling. A renal diet helps individuals manage their fluid intake, preventing extra fluid buildup and the associated stress on the kidneys.
- **Potassium and Phosphorus Control:** Elevated levels of potassium and phosphorus can be harmful to individuals with kidney disease. By managing the intake of these minerals, a renal diet prevents the stress on the kidneys caused by their inability to effectively excrete extra potassium and phosphorus.
- **Cardiovascular Health:** A renal diet also promotes cardiovascular health by controlling blood pressure and preventing heart-related complications. A healthy cardiovascular system is essential for reducing stress on the kidneys.
- **Delayed Dialysis or Transplantation:** For individuals with advanced kidney disease, adhering to a renal diet can slow the progression of the disease. This may delay the need for dialysis or kidney transplantation, reducing the overall stress on patients and providing a better quality of life.
- **Reduction of Complications:** Kidney disease can lead to various complications, including anemia, bone disease, and cardiovascular problems. A renal diet plays a significant role in preventing or minimizing these complications, further reducing the overall stress on individuals with kidney disease.

4. **Enhanced Quality of Life**

In addition to the physiological benefits, a renal diet can significantly enhance the quality of life for individuals with kidney disease. By addressing dietary challenges and managing symptoms, a renal diet contributes to a higher quality of life by:

- **Reducing Symptoms:** Symptoms such as fatigue, edema (swelling), and muscle weakness are common in kidney disease. By managing dietary restrictions and controlling complications, a renal diet can help alleviate these symptoms, providing patients with a better quality of life.
- **Regaining Control:** Living with a chronic health condition can be challenging, but a renal diet offers individuals a sense of control over their health. By following dietary guidance and adhering to nutritional principles, patients can actively participate in their care, making informed choices that positively impact their well-being.
- **Comfort and Well-Being:** Managing the dietary aspects of kidney disease enhances overall comfort and well-being. Patients often report feeling better, with increased energy levels and an improved sense of vitality when following a renal diet.
- **Increased Longevity:** By slowing the progression of kidney disease and reducing complications, a renal diet can contribute to a longer and healthier life. Delaying the need for dialysis or transplantation, improving cardiovascular health, and preventing complications all work together to increase longevity for patients with kidney disease.

CHAPTER 3: The Importance of Exercise for Renal

Kidney Health

Regular exercise is a crucial component of a holistic approach to maintaining and improving renal kidney health. While dietary modifications and medical treatments play a significant role in managing kidney disease, the benefits of exercise should not be overlooked.

Benefits of Exercise for Renal Kidney Health Staged-Based

1. **Improved Cardiovascular Health**

Cardiovascular health is crucial for individuals with kidney disease, as they often face an increased risk of cardiovascular complications. Exercise plays a significant role in improving cardiovascular health by:

- **Enhancing Circulation:** Regular physical activity improves blood flow and circulation, reducing the risk of cardiovascular problems such as heart disease, heart attacks, and strokes.
- **Lowering Blood Pressure:** Exercise helps lower blood pressure, which is a common complication in individuals with kidney disease. By reducing hypertension, exercise contributes to improved cardiovascular health and minimizes the risk of further kidney damage.
- **Strengthening the Heart:** Aerobic exercises like walking, jogging, or swimming strengthen the heart muscle, enhancing its ability to pump blood effectively throughout the body. This leads to improved overall cardiovascular function and reduced strain on the kidneys.
- **Managing Cholesterol Levels:** Regular physical activity helps maintain healthy cholesterol levels, reducing the risk of atherosclerosis and other cardiovascular complications commonly associated with kidney disease.

2. **Weight Management**

Maintaining a healthy weight is essential for individuals with kidney disease, as obesity can exacerbate the progression of the condition. Exercise contributes to weight management by:

- **Burning Calories:** Physical activity helps burn calories, contributing to weight loss or weight maintenance, depending on the individual's goals. This is vital for preventing obesity-related complications that can further strain the kidneys.
- **Improving Metabolism:** Frequent exercise boosts metabolism, enabling the body to burn calories more efficiently and sustain a healthy weight, which is advantageous for both overall health and kidney function.
- **Promoting Muscle Mass:** Strength training exercises promote muscle development, which can increase the body's resting metabolic rate and contribute to the maintenance of a healthy weight.

3. **Improved Muscle Strength and Endurance**

Maintaining muscle strength and endurance is essential for individuals with kidney disease, as it supports overall physical functionality and mobility. Exercise benefits muscle health by:

- **Preventing Muscle Wasting:** Regular physical activity, especially resistance training, helps prevent muscle wasting, a common concern in individuals with advanced kidney disease. Strengthening exercises can preserve muscle mass and improve overall muscle strength.
- **Enhancing Physical Function:** Improved muscle strength and endurance contribute to better physical function and mobility, letting individuals to perform daily activities with greater ease and independence.
- **Supporting Bone Health:** Strength training exercises not only strengthen muscles but also support bone health. This is particularly important for individuals with kidney disease, as they may be at an increased risk of bone-related complications.

4. **Better Blood Sugar Control**

Blood sugar management is crucial for individuals with diabetes-related kidney disease. Exercise plays a key role in controlling blood sugar levels by:

- **Enhancing Insulin Sensitivity:** Regular physical activity improves insulin sensitivity, enabling the body to use insulin more effectively and regulate blood sugar levels.
- **Promoting Glucose Utilization:** Exercise promotes the uptake of glucose by muscle cells, reducing the overall blood sugar levels in the body. This can help individuals with diabetes manage their condition more effectively.
- **Lowering the Risk of Type 2 Diabetes:** Regular exercise can aid in the prevention of type 2 diabetes for individuals at risk, consequently decreasing the likelihood of developing kidney disease associated with diabetes.

5. **Stress Reduction**

Chronic kidney disease can be emotionally and psychologically challenging for patients. Exercise can have a substantial impact on reducing stress levels through:

- **Releasing Endorphins:** Physical activity triggers the release of endorphins, neurotransmitters that promote feelings of well-being and reduce stress and anxiety, improving overall mental health.
- **Providing a Sense of Control:** Engaging in regular exercise empowers individuals with kidney disease, providing them with a sense of control over their health and well-being. This can significantly reduce the psychological burden of managing a chronic health condition.
- **Improving Sleep Quality:** Exercise can enhance sleep quality, a critical component of overall well-being and stress reduction. Adequate sleep contributes to better mental and emotional health, allowing individuals to cope more effectively with the challenges of kidney disease.
- **Boosting Mood:** Frequent physical activity can enhance mood and mitigate the risk of depression and anxiety, both of which are prevalent among individuals with chronic health conditions. This psychological boost can positively impact their ability to manage their kidney disease effectively.

It is important to recognize that individuals with renal kidney disease may progress through different stages of the condition, ranging from stage 1 to stage 4. The exercise guidelines should be tailored to the specific needs and limitations associated with each stage to ensure optimal benefits and safety.

Adapting Exercise Guidelines Based on Renal Health Stages

Stage 1: Early Kidney Disease

During the early stages of kidney disease, individuals may not exhibit significant symptoms, but preventive measures are crucial. Exercise recommendations for this stage may include:

- **Type of Exercise:** Focus on low-impact activities such as walking, cycling, or light aerobic exercises to promote cardiovascular health without placing excessive strain on the kidneys.
- **Frequency:** Aim for almost 150 mins of moderate-intensity exercise per week, distributed across multiple days.
- **Intensity:** Keep exercise intensity moderate, gradually increasing as tolerated.

Stage 2: Mild Kidney Disease

As kidney function begins to decline, adjustments in exercise routines become necessary:

- **Type of Exercise:** Continue with low-impact activities, but consider incorporating resistance training to maintain muscle mass.
- **Frequency:** Aim for a similar weekly exercise duration, but pay attention to individual tolerances and adjust accordingly.
- **Intensity:** Moderate intensity remains suitable, with attention to any signs of fatigue or discomfort.

Stage 3: Moderate Kidney Disease

With moderate kidney disease, exercise becomes a crucial component in managing overall health:

- **Type of Exercise:** Include a mix of cardiovascular exercises, resistance training, and flexibility exercises to address various aspects of health.
- **Frequency:** Aim for almost 150 mins of moderate-intensity exercise per week, with additional focus on strength training exercises 2-3 times a week.
- **Intensity:** Adjust intensity based on individual capabilities, with regular monitoring for any adverse effects.

Stage 4: Severe Kidney Disease

As kidney function further declines, exercise recommendations become more individualized:

- **Type of Exercise:** Emphasize low-impact activities and resistance training, with potential modifications based on specific health concerns.
- **Frequency:** Tailor exercise frequency based on individual capacity, with consideration for potential fatigue.
- **Intensity:** Low to moderate intensity is generally recommended, with careful attention to individual responses.

It's essential for individuals in all stages of kidney disease to consult with healthcare professionals and, if available, work with qualified exercise specialists to create personalized exercise plans that align with their specific health status and goals. Regular monitoring and adjustments to the exercise regimen will help ensure ongoing benefits while minimizing the risk of complications associated with kidney disease.

CHAPTER 4: Renal Diet Recipes

Breakfast Recipes

1. Apple Cinnamon Pancakes

Degree of difficulty: ★★★☆☆

Preparation time: 10 mins

Cooking time: 15 mins

Servings: 2

Ingredients:

- 1 teacup wheat flour
- 1 tbsp baking powder
- 1/2 tsp ground cinnamon
- 1/2 teacup unsweetened applesauce
- 1/2 teacup water
- 1 egg white
- 1/2 tsp vanilla extract

Directions:

1. Inside a container, blend the wheat flour, baking powder, and ground cinnamon.
2. Inside an extra container, whisk collectively the applesauce, water, egg white, and vanilla extract.
3. Place wet components into dry components and mix till well blended.
4. Warm non-stick griddle in a middling temp. and mildly oil it with cooking spray.
5. Pour ¼ teacup portions of batter onto the griddle to make pancakes.
6. Cook till bubbles form on the surface, then flip and cook the other side till golden brown.
7. Present with a spray of cinnamon.

Per serving: Calories: 220kcal; Fat: 1g; Carbs: 47g; Protein: 8g; Calcium: 180mg; Sodium: 280mg; Potassium: 190mg; Phosphorus: 220mg

2. Quinoa Breakfast Bowl

Degree of difficulty: ★★☆☆☆

Preparation time: 10 mins

Cooking time: 15 mins

Servings: 2

Ingredients:

- 1 teacup cooked quinoa
- 1/2 teacup fresh berries (e.g., blueberries, raspberries)
- 1/4 teacup severed almonds
- 1 tbsp honey (elective)

Directions:

1. Inside a container, blend the cooked quinoa, fresh berries, and severed almonds.
2. Spray with honey if anticipated.
3. Blend thoroughly and present.

Per serving: Calories: 280kcal; Fat: 10g; Carbs: 40g; Protein: 8g; Calcium: 80mg; Sodium: 5mg; Potassium: 240mg; Phosphorus: 140mg

3. Cottage Cheese with Pineapple

Degree of difficulty: ★☆☆☆☆

Preparation time: 5 mins

Cooking time: 0 mins

Servings: 2

Ingredients:

- 1 teacup low-fat cottage cheese
- 1 teacup fresh pineapple chunks

Directions:

1. Simply mix the low-fat cottage cheese with fresh pineapple chunks.
2. Present chilled.

Per serving: Calories: 160kcal; Fat: 2g; Carbs: 20g; Protein: 15g; Calcium: 160mg; Sodium: 320mg; Potassium: 180mg; Phosphorus: 200mg

4. *Mango Smoothie*

Degree of difficulty: ★☆☆☆☆

Preparation time: 5 mins

Cooking time: 0 mins

Servings: 2

Ingredients:

- 1 teacup fresh or frozen mango chunks
- 1 teacup low-fat yogurt
- 1/2 teacup unsweetened almond milk
- 1 tbsp honey (elective)

Directions:

1. Place mango chunks, low-fat yogurt, and unsweetened almond milk inside a mixer.
2. Blend till smooth.
3. If anticipated, include honey for extra sweetness.
4. Present cold.

Per serving: Calories: 150kcal; Fat: 2g; Carbs: 30g; Protein: 6g; Calcium: 250mg; Sodium: 80mg; Potassium: 400mg; Phosphorus: 150mg

5. *Veggie Omelet*

Degree of difficulty: ★★★☆☆

Preparation time: 10 mins

Cooking time: 10 mins

Servings: 2

Ingredients:

- 4 big egg whites
- 1/4 teacup bell peppers, cubed
- 1/4 teacup onions, cubed
- 1/4 teacup mushrooms, carved
- 1/4 teacup zucchini, grated
- 1/4 teacup low-fat cheese (elective)
- Salt and pepper as required

Directions:

1. In non-stick griddle, sauté the cubed bell peppers, onions, and mushrooms till soft.
2. Include grated zucchini then cook till wilted.
3. Inside a container, whisk the egg whites and a tweak of salt and pepper.
4. Pour egg solution into griddle with the vegetables.
5. Cook, lifting the edges to let uncooked eggs flow underneath, till the omelet is set.
6. If anticipated, spray with low-fat cheese and wrap the omelet in half.
7. Present hot.

Per serving: Calories: 120kcal; Fat: 3g; Carbs: 7g; Protein: 16g; Calcium: 80mg; Sodium: 230mg; Potassium: 300mg; Phosphorus: 120mg

6. *Oatmeal with Berries*

Degree of difficulty: ★☆☆☆☆

Preparation time: 2 mins

Cooking time: 5 mins

Servings: 2

Ingredients:

- 1 teacup rolled oats
- 2 teacups water
- 1/2 teacup mixed berries (e.g., strawberries, blueberries, raspberries)
- 1 tbsp honey (elective)

Directions:

1. Inside your saucepot, blend oats and water.
2. Cook in a middling temp., mixing irregularly, for 5 mins or 'til the oatmeal reaches your anticipated uniformity.
3. Split the oatmeal into two containers.
4. Top with mixed berries and a spray of honey if anticipated.

Per serving: Calories: 200kcal; Fat: 2g; Carbs: 40g; Protein: 6g; Calcium: 30mg; Sodium: 0mg; Potassium: 130mg; Phosphorus: 100mg

7. *Breakfast Burrito with Lean Turkey*

Degree of difficulty: ★★★☆☆

Preparation time: 10 mins

Cooking time: 10 mins

Servings: 2

Ingredients:

- 4 big egg whites
- 4 oz lean ground turkey
- 1/2 teacup bell peppers, cubed
- 1/2 teacup onions, cubed
- 1/2 tsp low-sodium taco seasoning
- 2 wheat tortillas

Directions:

1. In non-stick griddle, cook the lean ground turkey till browned.
2. Include cubed bell peppers and onions, sauté till soft.
3. Inside a container, whisk the egg whites and taco seasoning together.
4. Pour egg solution into griddle with the turkey and vegetables. Cook till the eggs are set.
5. Warm the wheat tortillas in a dry griddle or microwave.
6. Split egg solution among the tortillas, roll them up, and present.

Per serving: Calories: 250kcal; Fat: 6g; Carbs: 25g; Protein: 25g; Calcium: 60mg; Sodium: 300mg; Potassium: 300mg; Phosphorus: 200mg

8. *Pears with Ricotta Cheese*

Degree of difficulty: ★☆☆☆☆

Preparation time: 5 mins

Cooking time: 0 mins

Servings: 2

Ingredients:

- 2 ripe pears, carved
- 1/2 teacup low-fat ricotta cheese
- 2 tbsps honey
- Ground cinnamon for garnish

Directions:

1. Organize the pear slices on two plates.
2. Spoon a dollop of low-fat ricotta cheese over the pears.
3. Spray with honey then spray with ground cinnamon.
4. Present as a simple and delicious dessert or snack.

Per serving: Calories: 200kcal; Fat: 3g; Carbs: 40g; Protein: 7g; Calcium: 180mg; Sodium: 80mg; Potassium: 330mg; Phosphorus: 110mg

9. *Blueberry Muffins*

Degree of difficulty: ★★★☆☆
Preparation time: 15 mins
Cooking time: 20 mins
Servings: 2 (6 muffins)
Ingredients:

- 1 teacup wheat flour
- 1/4 teacup oat flour
- 1/4 teacup unsweetened applesauce
- 1/4 teacup rice milk
- 1/4 teacup fresh blueberries
- 2 tbsps honey
- 1/2 tsp baking powder
- 1/2 tsp baking soda

Directions:

1. Warm up your oven to 350 deg. F then line a muffin tin using paper liners.
2. Inside a container, blend the wheat flour, oat flour, baking powder, and baking soda.
3. Inside an extra container, mix the unsweetened applesauce, rice milk, and honey.
4. Blend wet & dry components, then wrap in the fresh blueberries.
5. Spoon the batter into the muffin teacups.
6. Bake for 20 mins or 'til a toothpick inserted into a muffin comes out clean.
7. Let cool prior to presenting.

Per serving: Calories: 220kcal; Fat: 2g; Carbs: 50g; Protein: 6g; Calcium: 50mg; Sodium: 250mg; Potassium: 200mg; Phosphorus: 160mg

10. *Waffle with Peach Compote*

Degree of difficulty: ★★☆☆☆
Preparation time: 10 mins
Cooking time: 10 mins
Servings: 2
Ingredients:

- 2 grain waffles
- 1 teacup carved peaches
- 1 tbsp honey
- 1/2 tsp cinnamon

Directions:

1. Toast the grain waffles till they are golden and crispy.
2. In small saucepan, heat the carved peaches, honey, and cinnamon at low temp. till warm.
3. Present the warm peach compote over the waffles.

Per serving: Calories: 240kcal; Fat: 2g; Carbs: 50g; Protein: 6g; Calcium: 60mg; Sodium: 240mg; Potassium: 260mg; Phosphorus: 140mg

11. *Chia Pudding with Berries*

Degree of difficulty: ★★☆☆☆
Preparation time: 5 mins
Cooking time: 0 mins
Servings: 2
Ingredients:

- 1/4 teacup chia seeds
- 1 teacup unsweetened almond milk
- 1/2 tsp vanilla extract
- 1/2 teacup mixed berries (e.g., strawberries, blueberries, raspberries)
- 1 tbsp honey (elective)

Directions:

1. Inside a container, blend chia seeds, unsweetened almond milk, and vanilla extract.
2. Stir well and allow it to relax for a couple of mins.
3. Stir again, cover, then put in the fridge for 2-4 hrs or overnight, mixing irregularly.
4. When ready to present, top using mixed berries and a spray of honey if anticipated.

Per serving: Calories: 170kcal; Fat: 8g; Carbs: 19g; Protein: 5g; Calcium: 260mg; Sodium: 100mg; Potassium: 160mg; Phosphorus: 130mg

12. *Breakfast Couscous*

Degree of difficulty: ★★☆☆☆
Preparation time: 10 mins
Cooking time: 5 mins
Servings: 2
Ingredients:

- 1 teacup wheat couscous
- 1 teacup boiling water
- 1/2 teacup fresh berries (e.g., blueberries, strawberries)
- 2 tbsps severed almonds
- 1 tbsp honey (elective)

Directions:

1. Place wheat couscous inside a heatproof container and pour the boiling water over it.
2. Cover and allow it to relax for 5 mins.
3. Fluff the couscous with a fork.
4. Top with fresh berries, severed almonds, and a spray of honey if anticipated.
5. Present warm.

Per serving: Calories: 320kcal; Fat: 6g; Carbs: 58g; Protein: 9g; Calcium: 50mg; Sodium: 10mg; Potassium: 240mg; Phosphorus: 150mg

13. Berry and Banana Smoothie Bowl

Degree of difficulty: ★★☆☆☆

Preparation time: 10 mins

Cooking time: 0 mins

Servings: 2

Ingredients:

- 1 teacup frozen mixed berries (e.g., blueberries, raspberries, strawberries)
- 1 ripe banana
- 1 teacup unsweetened almond milk
- 1/2 teacup plain Greek yogurt
- 2 tbsps honey (elective)
- 1/4 teacup wheat bran
- Fresh berries and carved banana for topping

Directions:

1. In your mixer, blend the frozen mixed berries, ripe banana, almond milk, Greek yogurt, and honey (if using). Blend till smooth.
2. Split the wheat bran among two containers.
3. Pour the smoothie solution over the wheat bran in every container.
4. Top with fresh berries and carved banana.
5. Present instantly and relish!

Per serving: Calories: 250kcal; Fat: 4g; Carbs: 48g; Protein: 9g; Calcium: 280mg; Sodium: 110mg; Potassium: 450mg; Phosphorus: 150mg

14. Greek Yogurt with Mixed Berries

Degree of difficulty: ★☆☆☆☆

Preparation time: 5 mins

Cooking time: 0 mins

Servings: 2

Ingredients:

- 1 teacup plain Greek yogurt
- 1 teacup mixed berries (e.g., blueberries, raspberries, strawberries)
- 2 tbsps honey (elective)
- 1/4 teacup wheat bran

Directions:

1. In two containers, divide the plain Greek yogurt.
2. Top the yogurt with mixed berries and spray with honey (if using).
3. Spray wheat bran over the top.
4. Present instantly as a healthy and delicious breakfast.

Per serving: Calories: 250kcal; Fat: 4g; Carbs: 40g; Protein: 15g; Calcium: 240mg; Sodium: 70mg; Potassium: 350mg; Phosphorus: 150mg

15. Homemade Wheat Bran Cereal

Degree of difficulty: ★★★☆☆
Preparation time: 15 mins
Cooking time: 0 mins
Servings: 2
Ingredients:

- 1 teacup wheat bran
- 2 teacups unsweetened rice milk
- 2 tbsps honey (elective)
- 1/2 teacup mixed berries (e.g., blueberries, raspberries, strawberries)

Directions:

1. Inside your saucepot, warm the rice milk in a middling temp. 'til warm but not boiling.
2. Stir in the wheat bran and continue to cook for a total of 5 mins, mixing irregularly, 'til the solution thickens.
3. Take out from temp. then stir in honey (if using).
4. Split the cereal into two containers.
5. Top with mixed berries.
6. Present warm and relish your homemade wheat bran cereal.

Per serving: Calories: 250kcal; Fat: 4g; Carbs: 45g; Protein: 10g; Calcium: 380mg; Sodium: 180mg; Potassium: 280mg; Phosphorus: 200mg

16. Zucchini and Carrot Pancakes

Degree of difficulty: ★★☆☆☆
Preparation time: 15 mins
Cooking time: 15 mins
Servings: 2
Ingredients:

- 1 zucchini, grated
- 1 carrot, grated
- 1/2 teacup wheat flour
- 1/2 tsp baking powder
- 1/4 teacup unsweetened almond milk
- 1 tbsp olive oil
- 1/2 tsp ground cumin
- Salt and pepper as required
- Fresh parsley for garnish

Directions:

1. Inside a big container, blend the grated zucchini and carrot.
2. Inside a distinct container, whisk collectively the wheat flour, baking powder, almond milk, olive oil, ground cumin, salt, and pepper.
3. Put the flour solution into the container with grated vegetables then stir till well blended.
4. Warm your non-stick griddle in a middling temp. and mildly oil it.
5. Spoon portions of the batter onto the griddle to form pancakes. Cook for 3-4 mins on all sides or 'til golden brown.
6. Present the zucchini and carrot pancakes garnished with fresh parsley.

Per serving: Calories: 230kcal; Fat: 8g; Carbs: 34g; Protein: 6g; Calcium: 120mg; Sodium: 220mg; Potassium: 350mg; Phosphorus: 150mg

17. Quinoa and Apple Porridge

Degree of difficulty: ★★☆☆☆

Preparation time: 10 mins

Cooking time: 15 mins

Servings: 2

Ingredients:

- 1 teacup quinoa, washed
- 2 teacups unsweetened almond milk
- 1 apple, skinned, cored, and cubed
- 1/2 tsp ground cinnamon
- 1 tbsp honey (elective)

Directions:

1. Inside your saucepot, blend the quinoa and almond milk. Boil, then decrease temp. then simmer for 10 mins, mixing irregularly.
2. Include the cubed apple and ground cinnamon to the quinoa solution. Continue to simmer for an extra 5 mins or 'til the quinoa is cooked and the porridge thickens.
3. Take out from temp. then stir in honey (if using).
4. Split the quinoa and apple porridge into two containers.
5. Present warm and relish!

Per serving: Calories: 320kcal; Fat: 6g; Carbs: 57g; Protein: 8g; Calcium: 320mg; Sodium: 90mg; Potassium: 450mg; Phosphorus: 200mg

18. Baked Pear with Cinnamon and Raisins

Degree of difficulty: ★★☆☆☆

Preparation time: 10 mins

Cooking time: 20 mins

Servings: 2

Ingredients:

- 2 ripe pears, divided and cored
- 1/2 tsp ground cinnamon
- 2 tbsps raisins
- 1 tbsp honey (elective)

Directions:

1. Warm up the oven to 350 deg.F.
2. Put the pear halves in your baking dish, cut side up.
3. Spray ground cinnamon uniformly across the pears.
4. Split the raisins among the pear halves, filling the cores.
5. Spray honey over the top (if using).
6. Cover the baking dish using foil and bake for 20 mins or 'til the pears are soft.
7. Present the baked pears warm, and relish this simple and flavorful dessert.

Per serving: Calories: 180kcal; Fat: 0.5g; Carbs: 46g; Protein: 1g; Calcium: 20mg; Sodium: 0mg; Potassium: 290mg; Phosphorus: 20mg

19. Blueberry and Lemon Yogurt Parfait

Degree of difficulty: ★☆☆☆☆

Preparation time: 10 mins

Cooking time: 0 mins

Servings: 2

Ingredients:

- 1 teacup plain Greek yogurt
- 1 teacup fresh blueberries
- 1 lemon, zested and juiced
- 2 tbsps honey (elective)
- 1/4 teacup granola
- Fresh mint leaves for garnish

Directions:

1. In two serving glasses or containers, layer the following: a spoonful of Greek yogurt, a handful of fresh blueberries, a spray of lemon zest, and a spray of lemon juice.
2. Replicate the layering till the glasses are filled.
3. Spray honey over the top (if using).
4. Finish by adding a layer of granola on the top.
5. Garnish with fresh mint leaves.
6. Present the Blueberry and Lemon Yogurt Parfait instantly.

Per serving: Calories: 250kcal; Fat: 5g; Carbs: 40g; Protein: 12g; Calcium: 260mg; Sodium: 80mg; Potassium: 180mg; Phosphorus: 150mg

20. Pineapple and Coconut Milk Rice

Degree of difficulty: ★★★☆☆

Preparation time: 10 mins

Cooking time: 20 mins

Servings: 2

Ingredients:

- 1 teacup long-grain white rice
- 1 1/2 teacups coconut milk (unsweetened)
- 1 teacup cubed pineapple (fresh or tinned in juice)
- 1/4 tsp ground ginger
- 2 tbsps honey (elective)

Directions:

1. Wash the rice thoroughly in cold water 'til the water runs clear.
2. Inside your saucepot, blend the washed rice, coconut milk, cubed pineapple, and ground ginger.
3. Boil the solution, then decrease the temp., cover, then simmer for 15-20 mins, or 'til the rice is soft then the liquid is immersed.
4. Fluff the rice with a fork and allow it to relax for a couple of mins.
5. Spray honey over the top (if using).
6. Present the Pineapple and Coconut Milk Rice as a flavorful side dish.

Per serving: Calories: 380kcal; Fat: 12g; Carbs: 63g; Protein: 5g; Calcium: 40mg; Sodium: 10mg; Potassium: 250mg; Phosphorus: 80mg

21. Carrot and Ginger Juice

Degree of difficulty: ★☆☆☆☆

Preparation time: 10 mins

Cooking time: 0 mins

Servings: 2

Ingredients:

- 4 big carrots, skinned and severed
- 1-inch piece of fresh ginger, skinned
- 1 tbsp lemon juice
- 2 tbsps honey (elective)
- Ice cubes (elective)

Directions:

1. Put the severed carrots and ginger in a juicer and extract the juice.
2. Stir in lemon juice & honey (if using) as required.
3. If anticipated, present the carrot and ginger juice over ice cubes.
4. Relish this refreshing and healthy drink!

Per serving: Calories: 100kcal; Fat: 0g; Carbs: 25g; Protein: 1g; Calcium: 60mg; Sodium: 120mg; Potassium: 590mg; Phosphorus: 40mg

Lunch Recipes

22. Turkey and Cranberry Sandwich

Degree of difficulty: ★☆☆☆☆

Preparation time: 10 mins

Cooking time: 0 mins

Servings: 2

Ingredients:

- 4 slices wheat bread
- 6 oz low-sodium roasted turkey breast
- 2 tbsps cranberry sauce
- 1/2 teacup fresh spinach leaves
- 1/4 teacup carved cucumber

Directions:

1. Place four pieces of your wheat bread on a flat surface.
2. On two of the slices, layer the roasted turkey breast, cranberry sauce, spinach leaves, and carved cucumber.
3. Top with your remaining bread slices to make sandwiches.
4. Cut in half if anticipated and present.

Per serving: Calories: 320kcal; Fat: 2g; Carbs: 45g; Protein: 25g; Calcium: 80mg; Sodium: 220mg; Potassium: 180mg; Phosphorus: 220mg

23. Baked Salmon with Lemon-Dill Sauce

Degree of difficulty: ★★☆☆☆

Preparation time: 10 mins

Cooking time: 20 mins

Servings: 2

Ingredients:

- 2 salmon fillets (6 oz. each)
- 1 lemon, carved
- 1 tbsp fresh dill, severed
- 1 tbsp olive oil
- Salt and pepper as required
- For the Lemon-Dill Sauce:
- 1/4 teacup plain Greek yogurt
- 1 tsp fresh lemon juice
- 1 tsp fresh dill, severed

Directions:

1. Warm up your oven to 375 deg.F.
2. Put salmon fillets on your baking sheet covered using parchment paper.
3. Spray olive oil over the salmon then flavour with salt, pepper, and severed dill.
4. Lay your lemon slices on top of the salmon.
5. Bake in to your warmed up oven for 20 mins or 'til the salmon flakes simply with a fork.
6. While salmon is baking, make the sauce by mixing lemon juice, yogurt, and dill in a small container.
7. Present the baked salmon with the lemon-dill sauce.

Per serving: Calories: 350kcal; Fat: 18g; Carbs: 5g; Protein: 40g; Calcium: 150mg; Sodium: 150mg; Potassium: 600mg; Phosphorus: 320mg

24. Caprese Salad with Balsamic Glaze

Degree of difficulty: ★☆☆☆☆

Preparation time: 10 mins

Cooking time: 0 mins

Servings: 2

Ingredients:

- 2 big ripe tomatoes, carved
- 1 teacup fresh mozzarella cheese, carved
- 1/4 teacup fresh basil leaves
- 2 tbsps balsamic glaze
- 1 tbsp extra-virgin olive oil
- Salt and pepper as required

Directions:

1. Organize tomato and mozzarella slices on a serving plate, follow one another.
2. Tuck fresh basil leaves among tomato and cheese slices.
3. Spray with balsamic glaze and olive oil.
4. Flavour using a tweak of salt and pepper.
5. Present instantly.

Per serving: Calories: 250kcal; Fat: 18g; Carbs: 7g; Protein: 14g; Calcium: 200mg; Sodium: 200mg; Potassium: 300mg; Phosphorus: 180mg

25. Zucchini Noodles with Pesto

Degree of difficulty: ★★☆☆☆

Preparation time: 15 mins

Cooking time: 5 mins

Servings: 2

Ingredients:

- 2 medium zucchinis, spiralized into noodles
- 1/4 teacup pesto sauce
- 2 tbsps grated Parmesan cheese (elective)
- Salt and pepper as required

Directions:

1. Warm a large griddle in a middling temp.
2. Include zucchini noodles then cook for 3-5 mins, shaking occasionally till they are fully heated and mildly soft.
3. Take out from temp. and shake with pesto sauce.
4. Flavour with salt and pepper as required.
5. If anticipated, spray with grated Parmesan cheese.
6. Present instantly.

Per serving: Calories: 250kcal; Fat: 20g; Carbs: 10g; Protein: 5g; Calcium: 80mg; Sodium: 180mg; Potassium: 600mg; Phosphorus: 80mg

26. Tuna Salad Wraps

Degree of difficulty: ★☆☆☆☆

Preparation time: 10 mins

Cooking time: 0 mins

Servings: 2

Ingredients:

- 1 tin (5 oz) low-sodium tuna, drained
- 1/4 teacup cubed celery
- 1/4 teacup cubed red onion
- 2 tbsps light mayonnaise
- 2 wheat tortillas
- 2 leaves of lettuce
- 1 small tomato, carved

Directions:

1. Inside a container, mix the drained tuna, cubed celery, cubed red onion, and light mayonnaise.
2. Lay out the wheat tortillas and place a lettuce leaf on each.
3. Split the tuna salad solution evenly among the two tortillas.
4. Top with tomato slices.
5. Roll up the tortillas, tucking in the sides as you go.
6. Slice in half and present.

Per serving: Calories: 300kcal; Fat: 10g; Carbs: 30g; Protein: 20g; Calcium: 80mg; Sodium: 220mg; Potassium: 220mg; Phosphorus: 160mg

27. Turkey and Vegetable Stir-Fry

Degree of difficulty: ★★☆☆☆

Preparation time: 15 mins

Cooking time: 15 mins

Servings: 2

Ingredients:

- 8 oz ground turkey
- 2 teacups mixed stir-fry vegetables (broccoli, bell peppers, snap peas, carrots)
- 2 tbsps low-sodium stir-fry sauce
- 1 tbsp vegetable oil
- 2 teacups cooked brown rice

Directions:

1. Inside a big griddle, warm vegetable oil over med-high temp.
2. Include ground turkey then cook till browned and fully cooked.
3. Take out the turkey from the griddle then put it away.
4. Inside the similar griddle, include the mixed stir-fry vegetables and stir-fry sauce. Cook for 5-7 mins till the vegetables are soft.
5. Return the cooked turkey to the griddle and blend.
6. Present the turkey and vegetable stir-fry over cooked brown rice.

Per serving: Calories: 400kcal; Fat: 12g; Carbs: 50g; Protein: 25g; Calcium: 60mg; Sodium: 350mg; Potassium: 450mg; Phosphorus: 220mg

28. Egg Salad Lettuce Wraps

Degree of difficulty: ★☆☆☆☆

Preparation time: 15 mins

Cooking time: 0 mins

Servings: 2

Ingredients:

- 4 hard-boiled eggs, severed
- 2 tbsps plain Greek yogurt
- 1 tbsp Dijon mustard
- 2 leaves of Bibb or butter lettuce
- 1/4 teacup cubed celery
- 1/4 teacup cubed red bell pepper
- Salt and pepper as required

Directions:

1. Inside a container, blend severed hard-boiled eggs, plain Greek yogurt, Dijon mustard, cubed celery, salt, and pepper.
2. Blend thoroughly.
3. Lay out 2 leaves of lettuce.
4. Split the egg salad solution uniformly among the lettuce leaves.
5. Top with cubed red bell pepper.
6. Roll up the lettuce leaves to make wraps.
7. Present instantly.

Per serving: Calories: 250kcal; Fat: 15g; Carbs: 10g; Protein: 18g; Calcium: 80mg; Sodium: 320mg; Potassium: 280mg; Phosphorus: 300mg

29. Grilled Shrimp and Asparagus

Degree of difficulty: ★★☆☆☆

Preparation time: 10 mins

Cooking time: 10 mins

Servings: 2

Ingredients:

- 8 oz big shrimp, that is skinned and deveined
- 1 bunch fresh asparagus
- 1 tbsp olive oil
- 1 piece garlic, crushed
- Zest and juice of 1 lemon
- Salt and pepper as required

Directions:

1. Warm up your grill to med-high temp.
2. Inside a container, mix olive oil, crushed garlic, lemon zest, lemon juice, salt, and pepper.
3. Shake the asparagus in the solution.
4. Thread shrimp onto skewers.
5. Grill the asparagus and shrimp for 3-4 mins on all sides till they are fully cooked and have grill marks.
6. Present hot.

Per serving: Calories: 200kcal; Fat: 9g; Carbs: 8g; Protein: 20g; Calcium: 80mg; Sodium: 150mg; Potassium: 400mg; Phosphorus: 200mg

30. Lentil Soup

Degree of difficulty: ★★☆☆☆

Preparation time: 10 mins

Cooking time: 30 mins

Servings: 2

Ingredients:

- 1 teacup dried green or brown lentils
- 4 teacups low-sodium chicken or vegetable broth
- 1/2 teacup cubed carrots
- 1/2 teacup cubed celery
- 1/2 teacup cubed onion
- 1 tsp olive oil
- 1/2 tsp dried thyme
- Salt and pepper as required

Directions:

1. Wash the lentils thoroughly.
2. Inside a big pot, warm olive oil in a middling temp. Include cubed onions, carrots, and celery. Sauté for 5 mins.
3. Include dried lentils, thyme, and broth.
4. Boil, decrease temp. then simmer for 25-30 mins, or 'til the lentils are soft.
5. Flavour with salt and pepper as required.
6. Present hot.

Per serving: Calories: 250kcal; Fat: 3g; Carbs: 45g; Protein: 17g; Calcium: 60mg; Sodium: 300mg; Potassium: 450mg; Phosphorus: 260mg

31. Grilled Chicken Salad

Degree of difficulty: ★★☆☆☆

Preparation time: 10 mins

Cooking time: 15 mins

Servings: 2

Ingredients:

- 2 boneless, skinless chicken breasts
- 4 teacups mixed greens (lettuce or kale)
- 1/2 cucumber, carved
- 1/2 red bell pepper, carved
- 1/4 teacup cherry tomatoes, divided
- 2 tbsps balsamic vinaigrette
- 1 tbsp olive oil
- Salt and pepper as required

Directions:

1. Warm up your grill or stovetop grill pan.
2. Flavour chicken breasts using a tweak of salt and pepper.
3. Grill the chicken for 6-7 mins on all sides or 'til fully cooked.
4. Inside a big container, blend the mixed greens, cucumber, red bell pepper, and cherry tomatoes.
5. Slice grilled chicken then place it on top of the salad.
6. Spray balsamic vinaigrette and olive oil over the salad.
7. Shake everything together carefully.
8. Present instantly.

Per serving: Calories: 300kcal; Fat: 10g; Carbs: 12g; Protein: 40g; Calcium: 60mg; Sodium: 120mg; Potassium: 400mg; Phosphorus: 220mg

32. Quinoa Stuffed Peppers

Degree of difficulty: ★★☆☆☆
Preparation time: 20 mins
Cooking time: 40 mins
Servings: 2
Ingredients:

- 2 big bell peppers, any color
- 1/2 teacup quinoa
- 1 teacup low-sodium vegetable broth
- 1/2 teacup black beans, that is drained and washed
- 1/2 teacup cubed tomatoes (tinned, no salt added)
- 1/4 teacup corn kernels (frozen or fresh)
- 1/4 teacup cubed onion
- 1/2 tsp chili powder
- Salt and pepper as required
- 1/4 teacup teared up low-sodium cheese (elective)

Directions:

1. Warm up your oven to 375 deg.F.
2. Cut tops off bell peppers then take out the seeds and membranes.
3. Inside your saucepot, blend quinoa and vegetable broth. Boil, then decrease temp., cover, then simmer for 15 mins or 'til quinoa is cooked.
4. Inside a distinct pan, sauté the cubed onion till it becomes luminous.
5. Inside a blending container, blend cooked quinoa, black beans, cubed tomatoes, corn, sautéed onion, chili powder, salt, and pepper.
6. Stuff bell peppers using the quinoa solution.
7. Put filled peppers in your baking dish and cover with foil.
8. Bake for 30 mins. Take out the foil then bake for an extra 10 mins till the peppers are soft.
9. If anticipated, top with teared up low-sodium cheese then bake for an extra 5 mins 'til the cheese is dissolved.

Per serving: Calories: 350kcal; Fat: 5g; Carbs: 65g; Protein: 15g; Calcium: 60mg; Sodium: 150mg; Potassium: 600mg; Phosphorus: 300mg

33. Sea Bass with Cilantro Pesto

Degree of difficulty: ★★★☆☆
Preparation time: 15 mins
Cooking time: 15 mins
Servings: 2
Ingredients:

- 2 sea bass fillets (6 oz each)
- 1 teacup fresh cilantro leaves
- 1/4 teacup almonds, toasted
- 1 piece garlic
- 2 tbsps olive oil
- Juice of 1 lime
- Salt and pepper as required

Directions:

1. Warm up your grill to med-high temp.
2. In blending container, blend fresh cilantro leaves, toasted almonds, crushed garlic, olive oil, lime juice, salt, and pepper. Blend till smooth to make the cilantro pesto.
3. Flavour the sea bass fillets using salt and pepper.
4. Grill the sea bass for 4-5 mins on all sides or 'til it flakes simply with a fork.
5. Present the grilled sea bass with a dollop of cilantro pesto on top.

Per serving: Calories: 300kcal; Fat: 20g; Carbs: 8g; Protein: 30g; Calcium: 100mg; Sodium: 100mg; Potassium: 500mg; Phosphorus: 300mg

34. Tofu and Vegetable Stir-Fry

Degree of difficulty: ★★☆☆☆

Preparation time: 15 mins

Cooking time: 15 mins

Servings: 2

Ingredients:

- 8 oz firm tofu, cubed
- 2 teacups mixed stir-fry vegetables (broccoli, bell peppers, snap peas, carrots)
- 2 tbsps low-sodium stir-fry sauce
- 1 tbsp vegetable oil
- 2 teacups cooked brown rice

Directions:

1. Inside a big griddle, warm vegetable oil in a med-high temp.
2. Include tofu cubes and stir-fry till mildly browned.
3. Take out tofu from the griddle then put it away.
4. Inside the similar griddle, include the mixed stir-fry vegetables and stir-fry sauce. Cook for 5-7 mins till the vegetables are soft.
5. Return the cooked tofu to the griddle and blend.
6. Present the tofu and vegetable stir-fry over cooked brown rice.

Per serving: Calories: 350kcal; Fat: 15g; Carbs: 40g; Protein: 15g; Calcium: 100mg; Sodium: 300mg; Potassium: 500mg; Phosphorus: 220mg

35. Chicken and Wild Rice Soup

Degree of difficulty: ★★☆☆☆

Preparation time: 15 mins

Cooking time: 30 mins

Servings: 2

Ingredients:

- 1 boneless, skinless chicken breast (6 oz)
- 1/2 teacup wild rice blend
- 4 teacups low-sodium chicken broth
- 1/2 teacup cubed carrots
- 1/2 teacup cubed celery
- 1/2 teacup cubed onion
- 1/2 tsp dried thyme
- Salt and pepper as required

Directions:

1. Inside a big pot, blend the chicken breast, wild rice, chicken broth, cubed carrots, celery, onion, dried thyme, salt, and pepper.
2. Boil, then decrease temp., cover, then simmer for 25-30 mins 'til the chicken is fully cooked and the rice is soft.
3. Take out chicken from the pot, shred it, and return it to the soup.
4. Present hot.

Per serving: Calories: 350kcal; Fat: 5g; Carbs: 45g; Protein: 30g; Calcium: 80mg; Sodium: 200mg; Potassium: 600mg; Phosphorus: 300mg

36. Roasted Vegetable Wrap

Degree of difficulty: ★★☆☆☆

Preparation time: 15 mins

Cooking time: 20 mins

Servings: 2

Ingredients:

- 2 grain tortillas
- 2 teacups mixed roasted vegetables (bell peppers, zucchini, eggplant, etc.)
- 1/2 teacup hummus
- 1/4 teacup feta cheese (elective)
- Fresh lettuce leaves
- Olive oil for drizzling
- Salt and pepper as required

Directions:

1. Warm up your oven to 425 deg.F.
2. Shake the mixed vegetables with a spray of olive oil, salt, and pepper.
3. Roast vegetables for 15-20 mins till they are soft and mildly caramelized.
4. Warm tortillas in a dry griddle for a min on all sides.
5. Disperse hummus on each tortilla.
6. Include a generous portion of roasted vegetables and some fresh lettuce leaves.
7. If anticipated, spray with feta cheese.
8. Roll up the tortillas and present.

Per serving: Calories: 350kcal; Fat: 12g; Carbs: 50g; Protein: 10g; Calcium: 150mg; Sodium: 250mg; Potassium: 600mg; Phosphorus: 150mg

37. Baked Cod with Herbs

Degree of difficulty: ★★☆☆☆

Preparation time: 10 mins

Cooking time: 20 mins

Servings: 2

Ingredients:

- 2 cod fillets (6 oz each)
- 2 tbsps fresh parsley, severed
- 1 tbsp fresh dill, severed
- 1 tbsp fresh chives, severed
- 1 lemon, finely carved
- 2 pieces garlic, crushed
- 1 tbsp olive oil
- Salt and pepper as required

Directions:

1. Warm up your oven to 375 deg.F.
2. Place cod fillets in a baking dish.
3. Inside a small container, mix severed parsley, dill, chives, crushed garlic, olive oil, salt, and pepper.
4. Disperse the herb solution uniformly across the cod fillets.
5. Lay lemon slices on top of cod.
6. Bake into your warmed up oven for 15-20 mins or 'til the cod flakes simply with a fork.
7. Present hot.

Per serving: Calories: 250kcal; Fat: 7g; Carbs: 5g; Protein: 40g; Calcium: 60mg; Sodium: 150mg; Potassium: 600mg; Phosphorus: 350mg

38. *Minestrone Soup*

Degree of difficulty: ★★☆☆☆
Preparation time: 15 mins
Cooking time: 30 mins
Servings: 2
Ingredients:

- 4 teacups low-sodium vegetable broth
- 1/2 teacup cubed carrots
- 1/2 teacup cubed celery
- 1/2 teacup cubed onion
- 1/2 teacup cubed zucchini
- 1/2 teacup cubed green beans
- 1/2 teacup low-sodium kidney beans, that is drained and washed
- 1/2 teacup cubed tomatoes
- 1/2 teacup wheat pasta (small shapes)
- 1/2 tsp dried oregano
- 1/2 tsp dried basil
- Salt and pepper as required
- Grated Parmesan cheese for garnish (elective)

Directions:

1. Inside a big pot, blend vegetable broth, cubed carrots, celery, onion, zucchini, green beans, kidney beans, cubed tomatoes, dried oregano, dried basil, salt, and pepper.
2. Boil, then decrease temp., cover, then simmer for 20-25 mins till the vegetables are soft.
3. Include pasta and cook according to its cooking time.
4. Present hot, garnished using grated Parmesan cheese if anticipated.

Per serving: Calories: 300kcal; Fat: 2g; Carbs: 60g; Protein: 12g; Calcium: 80mg; Sodium: 400mg; Potassium: 800mg; Phosphorus: 250mg

39. *White Fish soup*

Degree of difficulty: ★★★☆☆
Preparation time: 15 mins
Cooking time: 15 mins
Servings: 2
Ingredients:

- 2 white fish fillets (such as cod or haddock), around 6 oz. each
- 4 teacups fish or vegetable broth
- 1 small onion, finely severed
- 2 pieces garlic, crushed
- 1 medium carrot, cubed
- 1 celery stalk, cubed
- 1 small potato, skinned and cubed
- 1 tbsp olive oil
- 1 bay leaf
- Salt and pepper as required
- Fresh parsley or dill for garnish (elective)

Directions:

1. Inside a pot, warm olive oil over middling temp. Include the severed onion and sauté till luminous, then include crushed garlic and sauté for an extra min.
2. Pour in the fish or vegetable broth and raise it to a simmer.
3. Include the cubed carrot, celery, and potato to the simmering broth. Include the bay leaf and flavour with salt and pepper as required.
4. Gently place the white fish fillets into the simmering broth. Cover the pot and allow it to cook for around 8-10 mins or till the fish is fully cooked and flakes simply with a fork.
5. Take out the fish fillets from the soup and put them away. Take out the bay leaf from the broth.
6. Utilizing an immersion mixer or a regular mixer, carefully blend the soup till smooth.

7. Scoop the soup into containers and place the cooked fish fillets on top.

8. Garnish with fresh parsley or dill if anticipated, and present hot.

Per serving: Calories: 200kcal; Fat: 10g; Carbs: 20g; Protein: 25g; Calcium: 30mg; Sodium: 100mg; Potassium: 300mg; Phosphorus: 100mg

40. Baked Lemon Chicken

Degree of difficulty: ★★★☆☆
Preparation time: 10 mins
Cooking time: 30 mins
Servings: 2
Ingredients:

- 2 boneless, skinless chicken breasts
- 1 lemon, juiced and zested
- 1 tbsp olive oil
- 1 tsp dried thyme
- Salt and pepper as required
- 2 pieces garlic, crushed
- Fresh parsley for garnish

Directions:

1. Warm up the oven to 375 deg.F.
2. Inside a mini container, whisk collectively the lemon juice, lemon zest, olive oil, dried thyme, crushed garlic, salt, and pepper.
3. Put chicken breasts in your baking dish and pour the lemon solution over them.
4. Bake into your warmed up oven for 25-30 mins or 'til the chicken is fully cooked and the middle is no more pink in color.
5. Garnish with fresh parsley prior to presenting.

Per serving: Calories: 250kcal; Fat: 8g; Carbs: 4g; Protein: 40g; Calcium: 30mg; Sodium: 80mg; Potassium: 380mg; Phosphorus: 300mg

41. Cauliflower Fried Rice

Degree of difficulty: ★★☆☆☆
Preparation time: 15 mins
Cooking time: 15 mins
Servings: 2
Ingredients:

- 2 teacups cauliflower florets (riced cauliflower)
- 1/2 teacup cubed bell peppers
- 1/2 teacup cubed carrots
- 1/2 teacup frozen peas
- 2 tbsps low-sodium soy sauce
- 1 tbsp olive oil
- 1/2 tsp ground ginger
- 1/2 tsp garlic powder
- 2 green onions, severed
- Cooked and cubed chicken breast (elective)

Directions:

1. Inside your blending container, pulse the cauliflower florets till they resemble rice grains.
2. Warm olive oil in your large griddle in a med-high temp.
3. Include cubed bell peppers, carrots, and frozen peas. Stir-fry for 5-7 mins till vegetables are soft.
4. Include riced cauliflower, ground ginger, and garlic powder to the griddle. Stir-fry for an extra 5 mins.
5. Spray low-sodium soy sauce over the cauliflower solution then stir to blend.
6. If anticipated, include cooked and cubed chicken breast.
7. Garnish with severed green onions prior to presenting.

Per serving: Calories: 100kcal; Fat: 4g; Carbs: 14g; Protein: 4g; Calcium: 50mg; Sodium: 300mg; Potassium: 450mg; Phosphorus: 80mg

42. Mushroom and Pea Risotto

Degree of difficulty: ★★★☆☆
Preparation time: 10 mins
Cooking time: 30 mins
Servings: 2
Ingredients:

- 1 teacup Arborio rice (risotto rice)
- 1 teacup carved mushrooms
- 1/2 teacup frozen peas
- 1 small onion, finely severed
- 2 pieces garlic, crushed
- 4 teacups low-sodium vegetable broth
- 2 tbsps olive oil
- 1/4 teacup dry white wine (elective)
- 1/4 teacup grated Parmesan cheese (elective)
- Salt and pepper as required
- Fresh parsley for garnish

Directions:

1. Inside a huge saucepan, warm olive oil in a middling temp. Include severed onion and cook till luminous.
2. Include crushed garlic and carved mushrooms, and sauté till the mushrooms are browned.
3. Include Arborio rice then cook for a couple of mins, mixing regularly.
4. If using white wine, pour it into the pan then stir till it's mostly immersed.
5. Begin adding vegetable broth, one ladle at a time, mixing regularly then allowing the liquid to be immersed prior to including extra.
6. Continue this process till the rice is creamy and cooked to your anticipated uniformity (around 20-25 mins).
7. Stir in frozen peas then cook for an extra 2-3 mins.
8. If anticipated, stir in grated Parmesan cheese.
9. Flavour using salt and pepper as required.
10. Garnish with fresh parsley then present the Mushroom and Pea Risotto.

Per serving: Calories: 350kcal; Fat: 9g; Carbs: 60g; Protein: 7g; Calcium: 20mg; Sodium: 600mg; Potassium: 270mg; Phosphorus: 170mg

43. Butternut Squash Soup

Degree of difficulty: ★★☆☆☆
Preparation time: 15 mins
Cooking time: 25 mins
Servings: 2
Ingredients:

- 2 teacups cubed butternut squash
- 1 small onion, severed
- 2 pieces garlic, crushed
- 2 teacups low-sodium vegetable broth
- 1/2 tsp ground cinnamon
- 1/4 tsp ground nutmeg
- Salt and pepper as required
- 1 tbsp olive oil
- Greek yogurt (elective topping)
- Chopped chives (elective topping)

Directions:

1. Inside a huge pot, warm olive oil in a middling temp. Include severed onion and garlic and sauté till onion is luminous.
2. Include cubed butternut squash, ground cinnamon, and ground nutmeg. Cook for a couple of mins, mixing irregularly.
3. Pour in the low-sodium vegetable broth and raise to a boil.
4. Decrease temp., cover, then simmer for 20-25 mins or 'til the butternut squash is soft.
5. Utilize your mixer to puree the soup till smooth.
6. Flavour using salt and pepper as required.

7. Present the Butternut Squash Soup hot, and optionally top with a dollop of Greek yogurt and severed chives.

Per serving: Calories: 150kcal; Fat: 4g; Carbs: 30g; Protein: 2g; Calcium: 70mg; Sodium: 150mg; Potassium: 700mg; Phosphorus: 70mg

44. Chickpea and Cucumber Wrap

Degree of difficulty: ★★☆☆☆

Preparation time: 15 mins

Cooking time: 0 mins

Servings: 2

Ingredients:

- 1 tin (15 oz) chickpeas, that is drained and washed
- 1 cucumber, finely carved
- 1/2 teacup plain Greek yogurt
- 2 tbsps fresh dill, severed
- 2 wheat tortillas
- Salt and pepper as required
- Lettuce leaves for wrapping

Directions:

1. Inside your container, mash the chickpeas with a fork or potato masher till partially mashed.
2. Stir in plain Greek yogurt and fresh dill. Mix till well blended.
3. Flavour the chickpea solution using salt and pepper as required.
4. Lay out the wheat tortillas and disperse the chickpea solution evenly on each.
5. Top with cucumber slices and lettuce leaves.
6. Roll up the tortillas firmly, tucking in the sides as you go.
7. Slice each wrap in half and present the Chickpea and Cucumber Wrap.

Per serving: Calories: 320kcal; Fat: 7g; Carbs: 52g; Protein: 16g; Calcium: 150mg; Sodium: 410mg; Potassium: 370mg; Phosphorus: 190mg

Dinner Recipes

45. Seared Tofu with Ginger Glaze

Degree of difficulty: ★★☆☆☆

Preparation time: 10 mins

Cooking time: 10 mins

Servings: 2

Ingredients:

- 8 oz extra-firm tofu, cubed
- 2 tbsps low-sodium soy sauce
- 1 tbsp rice vinegar
- 1 tbsp honey
- 1/2 tsp fresh ginger, grated
- 1/2 tsp garlic, crushed
- 1 tsp vegetable oil
- Green onions for garnish (elective)

Directions:

1. Inside a container, blend the ginger, soy sauce, rice vinegar, honey, and garlic to make the glaze.
2. Warm vegetable oil in a non-stick griddle in a med-high temp.
3. Include tofu cubes then cook for 2-3 mins on all sides, or 'til they are golden brown.
4. Pour ginger glaze over the tofu then cook for an extra 1-2 mins, allowing the glaze to thicken and coat the tofu.
5. Garnish with carved green onions if anticipated.

Per serving: Calories: 230kcal; Fat: 8g; Carbs: 21g; Protein: 18g; Calcium: 220mg; Sodium: 350mg; Potassium: 260mg; Phosphorus: 180mg

46. Lemon Butter Shrimp

Degree of difficulty: ★★☆☆☆

Preparation time: 10 mins

Cooking time: 10 mins

Servings: 2

Ingredients:

- 8 oz large shrimp, that is skinned and deveined
- 2 tbsps unsalted butter
- 2 pieces garlic, crushed
- Juice of 1 lemon
- 1 tbsp fresh parsley, severed
- Salt and pepper as required

Directions:

1. Inside a big griddle, dissolve the butter in a middling temp.
2. Include crushed garlic and sauté for 1 min till fragrant.
3. Include shrimp then cook for 2-3 mins on all sides or 'til they turn pink and opaque.
4. Squeeze the lemon juice over the shrimp.
5. Flavour with salt, pepper, and severed parsley.
6. Stir to blend and present hot.

Per serving: Calories: 250kcal; Fat: 12g; Carbs: 3g; Protein: 30g; Calcium: 60mg; Sodium: 200mg; Potassium: 300mg; Phosphorus: 200mg

47. Lemon Dill Chicken

Degree of difficulty: ★★☆☆☆

Preparation time: 10 mins

Cooking time: 20 mins

Servings: 2

Ingredients:

- 2 boneless, skinless chicken breasts
- 1 lemon, juiced and zested
- 1 tbsp fresh dill, severed
- 1 piece garlic, crushed
- 1 tbsp olive oil

- Salt and pepper as required

Directions:

1. Inside a container, blend the lemon juice, lemon zest, severed dill, crushed garlic, and olive oil to make a marinade.
2. Flavour the chicken breasts using salt and pepper.
3. Pour marinade over the chicken and allow it to marinate for almost 10 mins.
4. Warm a griddle in a med-high temp. and include a touch of olive oil.
5. Cook chicken for 8 mins on all sides, or 'til it's fully cooked and the middle is no more pink in color.
6. Present hot, garnished with extra lemon zest and dill if anticipated.

Per serving: Calories: 220kcal; Fat: 9g; Carbs: 4g; Protein: 30g; Calcium: 40mg; Sodium: 90mg; Potassium: 370mg; Phosphorus: 260mg

48. Grilled Swordfish with Lemon Butter

Degree of difficulty: ★★★☆☆
Preparation time: 10 mins
Cooking time: 10 mins
Servings: 2
Ingredients:

- 2 swordfish steaks (6-8 oz each)
- 1 tbsp olive oil
- Juice of 1 lemon
- 2 tbsps unsalted butter
- 1 tsp fresh parsley, severed
- Salt and pepper as required
- Lemon wedges for garnish

Directions:

1. Warm up your grill to med-high temp.
2. Brush the swordfish steaks with olive oil then flavour with salt and pepper.
3. Grill the swordfish for 4-5 mins on all sides, or 'til it flakes simply with a fork.
4. In small saucepan, dissolve butter in a low heat. Stir in lemon juice and severed parsley.
5. Pour lemon butter sauce over the grilled swordfish.
6. Garnish with lemon wedges and present.

Per serving: Calories: 300kcal; Fat: 15g; Carbs: 2g; Protein: 35g; Calcium: 30mg; Sodium: 180mg; Potassium: 570mg; Phosphorus: 250mg

49. Turkey and Mushroom Risotto

Degree of difficulty: ★★★★☆

Preparation time: 10 mins

Cooking time: 30 mins

Servings: 2

Ingredients:

- 1 teacup Arborio rice
- 1/2 lb. ground turkey
- 2 teacups low-sodium chicken broth
- 1 teacup mushrooms, carved
- 1/2 onion, finely severed
- 1/2 tsp dried thyme
- 1/2 tsp garlic powder
- Salt and pepper as required
- 1 tbsp olive oil
- Fresh parsley for garnish (elective)

Directions:

1. Inside a big pan, warm the olive oil in a middling temp.
2. Include ground turkey then cook till browned, breaking it into small pieces.
3. Stir in the severed onion and mushrooms. Cook for 5 mins 'til the mushrooms are soft.
4. Include Arborio rice and for 2 mins.
5. Pour in ½ teacup of chicken broth and till immersed.
6. Continue adding the broth in 1/2 teacup increments, mixing regularly till the rice is creamy then cooked to your liking (around 20-25 mins).
7. Flavour using thyme, garlic powder, salt, and pepper.
8. Garnish with fresh parsley if anticipated.

Per serving: Calories: 400kcal; Fat: 10g; Carbs: 52g; Protein: 26g; Calcium: 40mg; Sodium: 350mg; Potassium: 300mg; Phosphorus: 250mg

50. Teriyaki Tofu with Steamed Broccoli

Degree of difficulty: ★★☆☆☆

Preparation time: 15 mins

Cooking time: 15 mins

Servings: 2

Ingredients:

- 8 oz extra-firm tofu, cubed
- 2 teacups broccoli florets
- 2 tbsps low-sodium teriyaki sauce
- 1 tbsp low-sodium soy sauce
- 1/2 tsp fresh ginger, crushed
- 1/2 tsp garlic, crushed
- 1 tsp vegetable oil
- Sesame seeds for garnish (elective)

Directions:

1. Steam the broccoli florets till they are soft-crisp, around 5-7 mins. Put away.
2. Inside a container, blend the teriyaki sauce, soy sauce, crushed ginger, and crushed garlic to make the marinade.
3. Warm the vegetable oil in a griddle in a med-high temp.
4. Include tofu cubes then cook for 2-3 mins on all sides till they are mildly browned.
5. Pour teriyaki marinade over the tofu and to cover.
6. Cook for an extra 2-3 mins, allowing the sauce to thicken and coat the tofu.
7. Present the teriyaki tofu with steamed broccoli and garnish with sesame seeds if anticipated.

Per serving: Calories: 220kcal; Fat: 9g; Carbs: 18g; Protein: 16g; Calcium: 200mg; Sodium: 500mg; Potassium: 480mg; Phosphorus: 240mg

51. Ratatouille with Rice

Degree of difficulty: ★★☆☆☆

Preparation time: 15 mins

Cooking time: 25 mins

Servings: 2

Ingredients:

- 1 small eggplant, cubed
- 1 zucchini, cubed
- 1 red bell pepper, cubed
- 1/2 onion, severed
- 1 tin (14 oz) low-sodium cubed tomatoes
- 2 pieces garlic, crushed
- 1 tsp dried basil
- 1 tsp dried oregano
- Salt and pepper as required
- 1 teacup cooked white rice
- Olive oil for sautéing

Directions:

1. Inside a big griddle, warm olive oil in a middling temp.
2. Include severed onion and garlic, and sauté for 2-3 mins till they become fragrant and mildly luminous.
3. Include cubed eggplant, zucchini, and red bell pepper. Sauté for an extra 5-7 mins till the vegetables start to soften.
4. Stir in the cubed tomatoes, dried basil, dried oregano, salt, and pepper.
5. Cover the griddle then simmer for 10-15 mins, or 'til the vegetables are soft and the flavors meld.
6. Present the ratatouille over cooked white rice.

Per serving: Calories: 320kcal; Fat: 6g; Carbs: 60g; Protein: 8g; Calcium: 70mg; Sodium: 400mg; Potassium: 750mg; Phosphorus: 180mg

52. Baked Chicken Breast with Herbs

Degree of difficulty: ★★☆☆☆

Preparation time: 10 mins

Cooking time: 25 mins

Servings: 2

Ingredients:

- 2 boneless, skinless chicken breasts
- 1 tsp olive oil
- 1/2 tsp dried thyme
- 1/2 tsp dried rosemary
- 1/2 tsp garlic powder
- Salt and pepper as required
- Lemon wedges (for garnish)

Directions:

1. Warm up your oven to 375 deg.F.
2. Place chicken breasts in a baking dish.
3. Spray them using olive oil then spray with thyme, rosemary, garlic powder, salt, and pepper.
4. Bake into your warmed up oven for 25 mins or 'til the chicken is fully cooked (internal temp. of 165 deg.F).
5. Present with lemon wedges for added flavor.

Per serving: Calories: 180kcal; Fat: 4g; Carbs: 0g; Protein: 35g; Calcium: 20mg; Sodium: 70mg; Potassium: 250mg; Phosphorus: 260mg

53. Grilled Pork Tenderloin

Degree of difficulty: ★★☆☆☆

Preparation time: 10 mins

Cooking time: 20 mins

Servings: 2

Ingredients:

- 1 pork tenderloin (about 1 lb.)
- 1 tsp olive oil
- 1/2 tsp dried thyme
- 1/2 tsp dried rosemary
- 1/2 tsp garlic powder
- Salt and pepper as required

Directions:

1. Warm up your grill to med-high temp.
2. Brush the pork tenderloin with olive oil then flavour it with thyme, rosemary, garlic powder, salt, and pepper.
3. Grill pork for 10 mins on all sides or 'til it reaches an internal temp. of 145 deg.F.
4. Take out from the grill, cover with foil, then allow it to rest for 5 mins prior to slicing.

Per serving: Calories: 220kcal; Fat: 5g; Carbs: 0g; Protein: 40g; Calcium: 10mg; Sodium: 70mg; Potassium: 480mg; Phosphorus: 340mg

54. Balsamic Glazed Salmon

Degree of difficulty: ★★★☆☆

Preparation time: 10 mins

Cooking time: 15 mins

Servings: 2

Ingredients:

- 2 salmon fillets (6-8 oz each)
- 2 tbsps balsamic vinegar
- 1 tbsp honey
- 1/2 tsp dried rosemary
- Salt and pepper as required
- Lemon wedges for garnish (elective)

Directions:

1. Warm up your oven to 375 deg.F.
2. Inside a small container, mix the salt, balsamic vinegar, honey, dried rosemary, and pepper to make the glaze.
3. Place salmon fillets in a baking dish.
4. Brush the salmon fillets with the balsamic glaze.
5. Bake into your warmed up oven for 12-15 mins or 'til the salmon flakes simply with a fork.
6. Garnish with lemon wedges if anticipated.

Per serving: Calories: 300kcal; Fat: 12g; Carbs: 10g; Protein: 35g; Calcium: 30mg; Sodium: 150mg; Potassium: 550mg; Phosphorus: 300mg

55. Quinoa and Chickpea Pilaf

Degree of difficulty: ★★☆☆☆

Preparation time: 10 mins

Cooking time: 20 mins

Servings: 2

Ingredients:

- 1 teacup quinoa, washed
- 1 tin (15 oz) low-sodium chickpeas, that is drained and washed
- 1/2 red bell pepper, cubed
- 1/2 small red onion, finely severed
- 1/2 tsp ground cumin
- 1/2 tsp ground coriander
- 1/4 tsp paprika
- 2 teacups low-sodium vegetable broth
- 1 tbsp olive oil
- Fresh cilantro for garnish (elective)

Directions:

1. Inside a big saucepan, warm the olive oil in a middling temp.
2. Include cubed red bell pepper and severed red onion. Sauté for 2-3 mins till softened.
3. Include quinoa and spices (cumin, coriander, and paprika). Stir for 1-2 mins.
4. Pour in vegetable broth then boil. Decrease temp., cover, then simmer for 15 mins, or 'til the quinoa is cooked and the liquid is immersed.
5. Stir in the chickpeas then cook for an extra 2-3 mins to heat through.
6. Garnish with fresh cilantro if anticipated.

Per serving: Calories: 320kcal; Fat: 7g; Carbs: 54g; Protein: 12g; Calcium: 60mg; Sodium: 200mg; Potassium: 340mg; Phosphorus: 200mg

56. Shrimp and Vegetable Kebabs

Degree of difficulty: ★★★☆☆

Preparation time: 20 mins

Cooking time: 10 mins

Servings: 2

Ingredients:

- 12 big shrimp, that is skinned and deveined
- 1 bell pepper, cut into chunks
- 1 zucchini, carved into rounds
- 1/2 onion, cut into wedges
- 1/4 teacup low-sodium teriyaki sauce
- 1 tbsp olive oil
- Wooden skewers, soaked in water

Directions:

1. Warm up your grill to med-high temp.
2. Thread the shrimp and vegetables onto the soaked wooden skewers, follow one another.
3. Inside a container, mix the low-sodium teriyaki sauce and olive oil to make a marinade.
4. Brush the kebabs with the marinade.
5. Grill the kebabs for 4-5 mins on all sides, or 'til the shrimp are pink and opaque.
6. Present hot.

Per serving: Calories: 200kcal; Fat: 7g; Carbs: 15g; Protein: 20g; Calcium: 60mg; Sodium: 420mg; Potassium: 450mg; Phosphorus: 200mg

57. Beef and Barley Soup

Degree of difficulty: ★★★☆☆

Preparation time: 15 mins

Cooking time: 1 hr

Servings: 2

Ingredients:

- 8 oz lean beef stew meat, cubed
- 1/2 teacup pearl barley
- 1 carrot, cubed
- 1 celery stalk, cubed
- 1/2 onion, severed
- 4 teacups low-sodium beef broth
- 1/2 tsp dried thyme
- Salt and pepper as required

Directions:

1. Inside a big pot, brown the beef cubes in a med-high temp.
2. Include severed onion, carrot, and celery. Sauté for 3-4 mins till the vegetables are mildly softened.
3. Stir in the pearl barley and dried thyme.
4. Pour in the low-sodium beef broth and raise the solution to a boil.
5. Decrease the temp., cover, then simmer for 45 mins to 1 hr, or 'til the beef is soft and the barley is fully cooked.
6. Flavour using salt and pepper and present hot.

Per serving: Calories: 350kcal; Fat: 8g; Carbs: 40g; Protein: 28g; Calcium: 60mg; Sodium: 450mg; Potassium: 720mg; Phosphorus: 220mg

58. Baked Eggplant Parmesan

Degree of difficulty: ★★★☆☆

Preparation time: 20 mins

Cooking time: 30 mins

Servings: 2

Ingredients:

- 1 medium eggplant, carved into 1/2-inch rounds
- 1 teacup low-sodium marinara sauce
- 1/2 teacup part-skim mozzarella cheese, teared up
- 1/4 teacup grated Parmesan cheese
- 1/2 tsp dried basil
- 1/2 tsp dried oregano
- Salt and pepper as required
- Olive oil cooking spray

Directions:

1. Warm up your oven to 375 deg.F.
2. Mildly salt your eggplant slices and let them sit for 10 mins to eliminate extra moisture. Pat them dry with a paper towel.
3. In baking dish, layer the eggplant slices, marinara sauce, and mozzarella cheese, then spray with dried basil, dried oregano, and grated Parmesan.
4. Replicate the layers till the entire components are utilized.
5. Finish using a layer of mozzarella and Parmesan on top.
6. Spray the top using olive oil cooking spray.
7. Bake into your warmed up oven for 25-30 mins, or 'til the cheese is bubbly and golden brown.
8. Let it cool for a couple of mins prior to presenting.

Per serving: Calories: 250kcal; Fat: 10g; Carbs: 25g; Protein: 15g; Calcium: 300mg; Sodium: 450mg; Potassium: 450mg; Phosphorus: 230mg

59. Turkey and Rice Casserole

Degree of difficulty: ★★☆☆☆

Preparation time: 15 mins

Cooking time: 30 mins

Servings: 2

Ingredients:

- 1 teacup cooked turkey, cubed
- 1 teacup cooked brown rice
- 1/2 teacup low-sodium chicken broth
- 1/2 teacup low-fat plain yogurt
- 1/4 teacup low-fat mozzarella cheese, teared up
- 1/4 teacup grated Parmesan cheese
- 1/2 tsp dried thyme
- Salt and pepper as required

Directions:

1. Warm up your oven to 375 deg.F.
2. Inside a container, blend the cooked turkey, cooked brown rice, low-sodium chicken broth, low-fat plain yogurt, and dried thyme. Blend thoroughly.
3. Flavour with salt and pepper as required.
4. Transfer solution to a oiled baking dish.
5. Spray low-fat mozzarella cheese and grated Parmesan cheese on top.
6. Bake into your warmed up oven for 25-30 mins, or 'til the casserole is fully heated and the cheese is bubbly and golden brown.
7. Present hot.

Per serving: Calories: 350kcal; Fat: 11g; Carbs: 31g; Protein: 30g; Calcium: 280mg; Sodium: 330mg; Potassium: 360mg; Phosphorus: 280mg

60. Lemon Herb Tilapia

Degree of difficulty: ★★☆☆☆

Preparation time: 10 mins

Cooking time: 15 mins

Servings: 2

Ingredients:

- 2 tilapia fillets
- 1 tbsp olive oil
- 1 lemon, juiced and zested
- 1 tsp dried basil
- 1 tsp dried parsley
- Salt and pepper as required

Directions:

1. Warm up your oven to 375 deg.F.
2. Place tilapia fillets in a baking dish.
3. Spray them using olive oil then spray with lemon juice, lemon zest, basil, parsley, salt, and pepper.
4. Bake into your warmed up oven for 15 mins or 'til the fish flakes simply with a fork.

Per serving: Calories: 150kcal; Fat: 6g; Carbs: 3g; Protein: 22g; Calcium: 20mg; Sodium: 60mg; Potassium: 250mg; Phosphorus: 190mg

61. Chicken and Artichoke Bake

Degree of difficulty: ★★☆☆☆

Preparation time: 15 mins

Cooking time: 35 mins

Servings: 2

Ingredients:

- 2 boneless, skinless chicken breasts
- 1 tin (14 oz) artichoke hearts, drained and quartered
- 1/2 teacup low-sodium chicken broth
- 1/4 teacup grated Parmesan cheese
- 2 pieces garlic, crushed
- 1/2 tsp dried oregano
- Salt and pepper as required
- Olive oil for greasing

Directions:

1. Warm up your oven to 375 deg.F.
2. Grease a baking dish with a small amount of olive oil.
3. Place chicken breasts in the baking dish then flavour with salt, pepper, and dried oregano.
4. Scatter the quartered artichoke hearts and crushed garlic around the chicken.
5. Pour chicken broth over the chicken and artichokes.
6. Spray your grated Parmesan cheese uniformly across the top.
7. Bake into your warmed up oven for 30-35 mins, or 'til the chicken is fully cooked.
8. Present hot with the pan juices.

Per serving: Calories: 320kcal; Fat: 9g; Carbs: 12g; Protein: 45g; Calcium: 250mg; Sodium: 480mg; Potassium: 580mg; Phosphorus: 350mg

62. Spaghetti Squash with Marinara

Degree of difficulty: ★★☆☆☆

Preparation time: 10 mins

Cooking time: 40 mins

Servings: 2

Ingredients:

- 1 small spaghetti squash
- 1 teacup low-sodium marinara sauce
- 1 tsp olive oil
- 1/2 tsp dried basil
- 1/2 tsp dried oregano
- Salt and pepper as required
- Grated Parmesan cheese for garnish (elective)

Directions:

1. Warm up your oven to 375 deg.F.
2. After cutting the spaghetti squash in half lengthwise, remove the seeds by scooping them out.
3. Brush cut sides with olive oil then flavour using salt and pepper.
4. Place squash halves cut-side down on your baking sheet then bake for 30-40 mins, or 'til the flesh can be simply scraped using a fork into "spaghetti" strands.
5. Inside your saucepot, heat the marinara sauce with dried basil and dried oregano.
6. Present the spaghetti squash with the marinara sauce on top. Garnish with grated Parmesan cheese if anticipated.

Per serving: Calories: 150kcal; Fat: 4g; Carbs: 30g; Protein: 3g; Calcium: 70mg; Sodium: 350mg; Potassium: 370mg; Phosphorus: 100mg

63. Garlic Lemon Chicken Breast

Degree of difficulty: ★★★☆☆

Preparation time: 10 mins

Cooking time: 25 mins

Servings: 2

Ingredients:

- 2 boneless, skinless chicken breasts
- 2 pieces garlic, crushed
- Zest and juice of 1 lemon
- 1 tbsp olive oil
- 1 tsp dried oregano
- Salt and pepper as required
- Fresh parsley for garnish

Directions:

1. Warm up the oven to 375 deg.F.
2. Inside a mini container, blend crushed garlic, lemon zest, lemon juice, olive oil, dried oregano, salt, and pepper.
3. Put the chicken breasts in your baking dish and pour the garlic lemon solution over them.
4. Bake in to your warmed up oven for 20-25 mins or 'til the chicken is fully cooked and the middle is no more pink in color.
5. Garnish with fresh parsley prior to presenting.

Per serving: Calories: 230kcal; Fat: 10g; Carbs: 3g; Protein: 30g; Calcium: 30mg; Sodium: 110mg; Potassium: 360mg; Phosphorus: 220mg

64. Vegetable Curry with Basmati Rice

Degree of difficulty: ★★★☆☆

Preparation time: 15 mins

Cooking time: 30 mins

Servings: 2

Ingredients:

- 1 teacup basmati rice
- 2 teacups water
- 1 tbsp olive oil
- 1 small onion, severed
- 2 pieces garlic, crushed
- 1 tsp curry powder
- 1/2 tsp ground turmeric
- 1/2 tsp ground cumin
- 1/2 tsp ground coriander
- 1 tin (15 oz) low-sodium chickpeas, that is drained and washed
- 1 teacup cubed mixed vegetables (e.g., bell peppers, zucchini, carrots)
- Salt and pepper as required
- Fresh cilantro for garnish

Directions:

1. Inside your saucepot, bring water to a boil, then include basmati rice. Decrease temp., cover, then simmer for 15-20 mins or 'til the rice is cooked.
2. Inside a huge griddle, warm olive oil in a middling temp. Include severed onion and garlic and sauté till onion is luminous.
3. Include curry powder, ground turmeric, ground cumin, and ground coriander to the griddle. Stir for a min till fragrant.
4. Stir in chickpeas, and cubed mixed vegetables.
5. Simmer for 10-15 mins till the vegetables are soft.
6. Flavour using salt and pepper as required.
7. Present the Vegetable Curry over cooked basmati rice, garnished with fresh cilantro.

Per serving: Calories: 220kcal; Fat: 5g; Carbs: 38g; Protein: 8g; Calcium: 90mg; Sodium: 340mg; Potassium: 500mg; Phosphorus: 150mg

65. *Cauliflower Steak with Herb Sauce*

Degree of difficulty: ★★★☆☆
Preparation time: 15 mins
Cooking time: 20 mins
Servings: 2
Ingredients:

- 1 big cauliflower head
- 2 tbsps olive oil
- Salt and pepper as required
- For the Herb Sauce:
- 1/2 teacup plain Greek yogurt
- 1/4 teacup fresh parsley, severed
- 1/4 teacup fresh cilantro, severed
- Zest and juice of 1 lemon
- 1 piece garlic, crushed
- Salt and pepper as required

Directions:

1. Warm up the oven to 425 deg.F.
2. Trim the leaves & stem of the cauliflower, leaving the core intact. Slice the cauliflower into two 1-inch thick "steaks."
3. Brush both sides of the cauliflower steaks using olive oil and flavour using salt and pepper.
4. Put the cauliflower steaks on a baking sheet and roast into your warmed up oven for 20 mins or 'til they are soft and browned.
5. While cauliflower is roasting, prepare the herb sauce. Inside a container, blend plain Greek yogurt, severed fresh parsley, severed fresh cilantro, lemon zest, lemon juice, crushed garlic, salt, and pepper.
6. Present the Cauliflower Steak with the Herb Sauce sprayed on top.

Per serving: Calories: 100kcal; Fat: 7g; Carbs: 8g; Protein: 4g; Calcium: 50mg; Sodium: 80mg; Potassium: 500mg; Phosphorus: 100mg

66. *Lentil Bolognese with Wheat Pasta*

Degree of difficulty: ★★☆☆☆
Preparation time: 15 mins
Cooking time: 25 mins
Servings: 2
Ingredients:

- 1 teacup dried brown lentils, that is washed and drained
- 2 teacups low-sodium vegetable broth
- 1/2 onion, severed
- 2 pieces garlic, crushed
- 1 carrot, cubed
- 1 celery stalk, cubed
- 1 tsp dried basil
- 1 tsp dried oregano
- Salt and pepper as required
- 4 oz. wheat pasta (of your choice)
- Fresh basil leaves for garnish (elective)

Directions:

1. Inside a huge pot, blend lentils, low-sodium vegetable broth, severed onion, crushed garlic, cubed carrot, and cubed celery.
2. Boil, then decrease temp. and simmer for 20-25 mins or 'til lentils are soft and most of the liquid is immersed.
3. Stir in dried basil, dried oregano, salt, and pepper. Simmer for an extra 5-10 mins.
4. While the lentil Bolognese is simmering, cook the wheat pasta as per to the package guidelines.
5. Present the lentil Bolognese over cooked wheat pasta, garnished with fresh basil leaves if anticipated.

Per serving: Calories: 400kcal; Fat: 2g; Carbs: 78g; Protein: 22g; Calcium: 70mg; Sodium: 170mg; Potassium: 354mg; Phosphorus: 280mg

67. *Vegetable and Bean Chili*

Degree of difficulty: ★★☆☆☆

Preparation time: 15 mins

Cooking time: 30 mins

Servings: 2

Ingredients:

- 1 tin (15 oz) low-sodium kidney beans, that is drained and washed
- 1 tin (15 oz) low-sodium black beans, that is drained and washed
- 1 teacup cubed mixed vegetables (e.g., bell peppers, zucchini, corn)
- 1/2 onion, severed
- 2 pieces garlic, crushed
- 1 tbsp chili powder
- 1 tsp ground cumin
- Salt and pepper as required
- Chopped cilantro for garnish (elective)

Directions:

1. Inside a huge pot, warm olive oil in a middling temp. Include severed onion and crushed garlic and sauté till onion is luminous.
2. Include cubed mixed vegetables and sauté for a couple of mins.
3. Stir in kidney beans, black beans, chili powder, ground cumin, salt, and pepper.
4. Simmer for 20-25 mins or 'til the vegetables are soft.
5. Present the Vegetable and Bean Chili hot, garnished with severed cilantro if anticipated.

Per serving: Calories: 320kcal; Fat: 1g; Carbs: 60g; Protein: 17g; Calcium: 110mg; Sodium: 300mg; Potassium: 750mg; Phosphorus: 250mg

68. *Mixed Green Salad with Lemon Vinaigrette*

Degree of difficulty: ★☆☆☆☆

Preparation time: 10 mins

Cooking time: 0 mins

Servings: 2

Ingredients:

- 4 teacups mixed salad greens
- 1/2 cucumber, carved
- 1/2 bell pepper, finely carved
- 1/4 red onion, finely carved
  For the Lemon Vinaigrette:
- Juice and zest of 1 lemon
- 2 tbsps olive oil
- 1 tsp Dijon mustard
- Salt and pepper as required

Directions:

1. Inside a huge salad container, blend mixed salad greens, carved cucumber, carved bell pepper, and finely carved red onion.
2. Inside a mini container, whisk collectively lemon juice, lemon zest, olive oil, Dijon mustard, salt, and pepper to make the vinaigrette.
3. Spray the lemon vinaigrette over the salad then shake to cover.
4. Present the Mixed Green Salad as a refreshing side dish.

Per serving: Calories: 120kcal; Fat: 10g; Carbs: 8g; Protein: 2g; Calcium: 40mg; Sodium: 20mg; Potassium: 280mg; Phosphorus: 50mg

69. Arugula and Pear Salad

Degree of difficulty: ★☆☆☆☆

Preparation time: 10 mins

Cooking time: 0 mins

Servings: 2

Ingredients:

- 4 teacups arugula
- 1 ripe pear, finely carved
- 1/4 teacup severed walnuts
- For the Lemon Vinaigrette
- Juice and zest of 1 lemon
- 2 tbsps olive oil
- 1 tsp Dijon mustard
- Salt and pepper as required

Directions:

1. Inside a huge salad container, blend arugula, finely carved pear, and severed walnuts.

2. Inside a mini container, whisk collectively lemon juice, lemon zest, olive oil, Dijon mustard, salt, and pepper to make the vinaigrette.

3. Spray the lemon vinaigrette over the salad then shake to cover.

4. Present the Arugula and Pear Salad for a delightful and nutritious side dish.

Per serving: Calories: 160kcal; Fat: 14g; Carbs: 8g; Protein: 2g; Calcium: 80mg; Sodium: 20mg; Potassium: 260mg; Phosphorus: 40mg

Salad Recipes

70. Roasted Beet Salad

Degree of difficulty: ★★★☆☆

Preparation time: 15 mins

Cooking time: 45 mins

Servings: 2

Ingredients:

- 2 medium-sized beets, roasted, skinned, and cubed
- 2 teacups mixed greens (e.g. arugula)
- 1/4 teacup crumbled goat cheese
- 2 tbsps balsamic vinaigrette dressing
- 2 tbsps severed walnuts (elective)

Directions:

1. Warm up the oven to 400 deg.F. Wrap beets in foil then roast for 45 mins or 'til soft. Let them cool, then peel and dice.
2. Organize mixed greens on two plates and top with roasted beets and crumbled goat cheese.
3. Spray balsamic vinaigrette dressing over the salad then spray with severed walnuts if anticipated.

Per serving: Calories: 220kcal; Fat: 14g; Carbs: 18g; Protein: 7g; Calcium: 80mg; Sodium: 60mg; Potassium: 600mg; Phosphorus: 150mg

71. Pear and Walnut Salad

Degree of difficulty: ★☆☆☆☆

Preparation time: 10 mins

Cooking time: 0 mins

Servings: 2

Ingredients:

- 2 teacups mixed greens
- 1 ripe pear, finely carved
- 1/4 teacup severed walnuts
- 2 tbsps olive oil
- 2 tbsps balsamic vinegar
- 1 tsp honey
- Salt and pepper as required

Directions:

1. Inside a big container, blend mixed greens, carved pear, and severed walnuts.
2. Inside a small container, whisk collectively your olive oil, balsamic vinegar, honey, salt, and pepper.
3. Afterwards, drizzle the dressing across the salad. and shake carefully to cover.

Per serving: Calories: 280kcal; Fat: 21g; Carbs: 21g; Protein: 3g; Calcium: 30mg; Sodium: 20mg; Potassium: 220mg; Phosphorus: 70mg

72. Mixed Greens with Raspberry Vinaigrette

Degree of difficulty: ★☆☆☆☆

Preparation time: 10 mins

Cooking time: 0 mins

Servings: 2

Ingredients:

- 4 teacups mixed greens
- 1/2 teacup fresh raspberries
- 2 tbsps olive oil
- 2 tbsps balsamic vinegar
- 1 tsp honey
- Salt and pepper as required

Directions:

1. Inside a big container, blend mixed greens and fresh raspberries.
2. Inside a distinct container, whisk collectively olive oil, balsamic vinegar, honey, salt, and pepper.
3. Transfer raspberry vinaigrette over the salad and shake carefully to cover.

Per serving: Calories: 180kcal; Fat: 14g; Carbs: 14g; Protein: 2g; Calcium: 50mg; Sodium: 20mg; Potassium: 180mg; Phosphorus: 40mg

73. Lentil and Vegetable Salad

Degree of difficulty: ★★☆☆☆

Preparation time: 20 mins

Cooking time: 20 mins

Servings: 2

Ingredients:

- 1/2 teacup dried green or brown lentils
- 1 teacup water
- 1 teacup cubed mixed vegetables (e.g., bell peppers, carrots, and zucchini)
- 2 tbsps olive oil
- 2 tbsps red wine vinegar
- 1 piece garlic, crushed
- 1/4 tsp dried oregano
- Salt and pepper as required

Directions:

1. Wash the lentils and put them in a saucepan with 1 teacup of water. Boil, then decrease the temp., cover, then simmer for 20 mins or 'til the lentils are soft. Drain any extra water.
2. Inside a big container, blend the cooked lentils and cubed mixed vegetables.
3. Inside a small container, whisk collectively crushed garlic, olive oil, red wine vinegar, and dried oregano.
4. Afterwards, drizzle the dressing across the salad. and shake to blend. Flavour with salt and pepper.

Per serving: Calories: 300kcal; Fat: 12g; Carbs: 38g; Protein: 12g; Calcium: 50mg; Sodium: 10mg; Potassium: 450mg; Phosphorus: 180mg

74. Spinach and Strawberry Salad

Degree of difficulty: ★☆☆☆☆

Preparation time: 10 mins

Cooking time: 0 mins

Servings: 2

Ingredients:

- 2 teacups fresh spinach leaves
- 1 teacup carved strawberries
- 2 tbsps balsamic vinaigrette dressing
- 1/4 teacup crumbled feta cheese
- 2 tbsps severed walnuts (elective)

Directions:

1. Wash and dry the spinach leaves and strawberries.
2. Inside a big container, blend the spinach and strawberries.
3. Spray balsamic vinaigrette dressing over salad and shake carefully.
4. Top with crumbled feta cheese and severed walnuts if anticipated.

Per serving: Calories: 150kcal; Fat: 7g; Carbs: 17g; Protein: 5g; Calcium: 120mg; Sodium: 80mg; Potassium: 270mg; Phosphorus: 80mg

75. Quinoa and Black Bean Salad

Degree of difficulty: ★★☆☆☆

Preparation time: 20 mins

Cooking time: 15 mins

Servings: 2

Ingredients:

- 1/2 teacup quinoa, washed
- 1 teacup water
- 1 tin (15 oz) low-sodium black beans, that is drained and washed
- 1/2 teacup cubed red bell pepper
- 1/4 teacup severed fresh cilantro
- 2 tbsps olive oil
- 2 tbsps fresh lime juice
- 1 tsp ground cumin
- Salt and pepper as required

Directions:

1. Inside medium saucepot, boil the water and include quinoa. Decrease temp., cover, then simmer for 15 mins, or 'til quinoa is soft and water is immersed. Take from temp. then fluff with a fork.
2. Inside a big container, blend cooked quinoa, black beans, red bell pepper, and cilantro.
3. Inside a small container, whisk collectively your lime juice, olive oil, and ground cumin.
4. Afterwards, drizzle the dressing across the salad. and shake to blend. Flavour with salt and pepper.

Per serving: Calories: 370kcal; Fat: 13g; Carbs: 55g; Protein: 12g; Calcium: 60mg; Sodium: 20mg; Potassium: 430mg; Phosphorus: 160mg

76. Chicken Caesar Salad

Degree of difficulty: ★★☆☆☆

Preparation time: 15 mins

Cooking time: 15 mins

Servings: 2

Ingredients:

- 2 boneless, skinless chicken breasts
- 4 teacups romaine lettuce, severed
- 1/4 teacup grated Parmesan cheese
- 4 tbsps Caesar dressing
- Croutons

Directions:

1. Flavour chicken breasts using salt and pepper, then grill or pan-sear till fully cooked. Slice into thin strips.
2. Inside a big container, blend severed romaine lettuce, grated Parmesan cheese, and chicken strips.
3. Transfer Caesar dressing over the salad and shake to cover.
4. Top with croutons if anticipated.

Per serving: Calories: 320kcal; Fat: 17g; Carbs: 6g; Protein: 32g; Calcium: 120mg; Sodium: 160mg; Potassium: 420mg; Phosphorus: 280mg

77. Chickpea Salad

Degree of difficulty: ★★☆☆☆

Preparation time: 15 mins

Cooking time: 0 mins

Servings: 2

Ingredients:

- 1 tin (15 oz) low-sodium chickpeas, that is drained and washed
- 1/2 teacup cubed cucumber
- 1/2 teacup cubed red bell pepper
- 1/4 teacup cubed red onion
- 2 tbsps fresh lemon juice
- 2 tbsps olive oil
- 2 tbsps fresh parsley, severed
- Salt and pepper as required

Directions:

1. Inside a big container, blend chickpeas, cucumber, red bell pepper, and red onion.
2. Inside a small container, whisk collectively your olive oil, lemon juice, and severed parsley.
3. Afterwards, drizzle the dressing across the salad. and shake to blend.
4. Flavour with salt and pepper as required.

Per serving: Calories: 310kcal; Fat: 14g; Carbs: 39g; Protein: 11g; Calcium: 60mg; Sodium: 20mg; Potassium: 350mg; Phosphorus: 80mg

78. Roasted Red Pepper Salad

Degree of difficulty: ★★☆☆☆

Preparation time: 15 mins

Cooking time: 0 mins

Servings: 2

Ingredients:

- 2 big roasted red peppers, carved into strips
- 1/2 teacup carved black olives
- 1/4 teacup crumbled feta cheese
- 2 tbsps olive oil
- 2 tbsps balsamic vinegar
- 1 tsp dried basil
- Salt and pepper as required

Directions:

1. Inside a container, blend roasted red pepper strips, carved black olives, and crumbled feta cheese.
2. Inside a small container, whisk collectively your olive oil, balsamic vinegar, dried basil, salt, and pepper.
3. Afterwards, drizzle the dressing across the salad. and shake carefully to cover.

Per serving: Calories: 230kcal; Fat: 18g; Carbs: 12g; Protein: 4g; Calcium: 100mg; Sodium: 150mg; Potassium: 300mg; Phosphorus: 70mg

79. Greek Cucumber Salad

Degree of difficulty: ★★☆☆☆

Preparation time: 15 mins

Cooking time: 0 mins

Servings: 2

Ingredients:

- 1 cucumber, cubed
- 1 teacup cherry tomatoes, divided
- 1/2 teacup cubed red onion
- 1/4 teacup crumbled feta cheese
- 2 tbsps olive oil
- 2 tbsps fresh lemon juice
- 1 tsp dried oregano
- Salt and pepper as required

Directions:

1. Inside a container, blend cucumber, cherry tomatoes, and red onion.
2. Inside a small container, whisk collectively your olive oil, lemon juice, and oregano.
3. Afterwards, drizzle the dressing across the salad. and shake to blend.
4. Top with crumbled feta cheese then flavour with salt and pepper.

Per serving: Calories: 220kcal; Fat: 18g; Carbs: 11g; Protein: 4g; Calcium: 120mg; Sodium: 90mg; Potassium: 330mg; Phosphorus: 70mg

80. Asian Cabbage Salad

Degree of difficulty: ★★☆☆☆
Preparation time: 15 mins
Cooking time: 0 mins
Servings: 2
Ingredients:

- 3 teacups teared up Napa cabbage
- 1 teacup teared up carrots
- 1/4 teacup carved green onions
- 2 tbsps low-sodium soy sauce
- 2 tbsps rice vinegar
- 1 tbsp sesame oil
- 1 tsp honey
- 1/4 teacup severed fresh cilantro (elective)

Directions:

1. Inside a big container, blend teared up Napa cabbage, teared up carrots, and carved green onions.
2. Inside a distinct container, whisk collectively low-sodium soy sauce, rice vinegar, sesame oil, and honey.
3. Afterwards, drizzle the dressing across the salad. and shake to blend. Include severed cilantro if anticipated.

Per serving: Calories: 150kcal; Fat: 7g; Carbs: 17g; Protein: 3g; Calcium: 70mg; Sodium: 250mg; Potassium: 300mg; Phosphorus: 70mg

81. Tofu and Edamame Salad

Degree of difficulty: ★★☆☆☆
Preparation time: 15 mins
Cooking time: 5 mins (for tofu)
Servings: 2
Ingredients:

- 8 oz firm tofu, cubed
- 1 teacup shelled edamame, cooked and cooled
- 4 teacups mixed greens
- 2 tbsps low-sodium soy sauce
- 2 tbsps rice vinegar
- 1 tbsp sesame oil
- 1/2 tsp ginger, crushed
- 1/2 tsp garlic, crushed
- Salt and pepper as required

Directions:

1. In non-stick pan, sauté tofu cubes in a middling temp. 'til they are mildly browned on all sides. Put away to cool.
2. Inside a big container, blend mixed greens, cooked edamame, and tofu.
3. Inside a distinct container, whisk collectively low-sodium soy sauce, rice vinegar, sesame oil, ginger, garlic, salt, and pepper.
4. Afterwards, drizzle the dressing across the salad. and shake carefully to cover.

Per serving: Calories: 300kcal; Fat: 16g; Carbs: 17g; Protein: 24g; Calcium: 160mg; Sodium: 310mg; Potassium: 570mg; Phosphorus: 340mg

82. Caesar Salad with Croutons

Degree of difficulty: ★★☆☆☆

Preparation time: 15 mins

Cooking time: 5 mins (for croutons)

Servings: 2

Ingredients:

- 4 teacups romaine lettuce, severed
- 1/4 teacup grated Parmesan cheese
- 2 tbsps low-sodium Caesar dressing
- 2 slices grain bread, cubed (for croutons)
- 1 tbsp olive oil (for croutons)
- Salt and pepper as required

Directions:

1. Inside a big container, blend severed romaine lettuce and grated Parmesan cheese.
2. Inside a small container, mix low-sodium Caesar dressing with salt and pepper as required.
3. Shake the dressing over the salad.
4. To make croutons, warm olive oil in a pan, include bread cubes, then cook till they are crisp and golden. Let cool prior to adding to the salad.

Per serving: Calories: 270kcal; Fat: 18g; Carbs: 15g; Protein: 10g; Calcium: 120mg; Sodium: 210mg; Potassium: 180mg; Phosphorus: 160mg

83. Citrus Salad with Almonds

Degree of difficulty: ★☆☆☆☆

Preparation time: 10 mins

Cooking time: 0 mins

Servings: 2

Ingredients:

- 4 tangerines, skinned and carved
- 1 grapefruit, skinned and carved
- 2 tbsps carved almonds
- 2 tbsps honey
- 1/2 tsp ground cinnamon
- Fresh mint leaves for garnish (elective)

Directions:

1. Organize the carved tangerines and grapefruit on two plates.
2. Spray carved almonds over the citrus slices.
3. Inside a small container, mix honey and ground cinnamon.
4. Spray honey-cinnamon solution over the fruit and garnish with fresh mint leaves if anticipated.

Per serving: Calories: 250kcal; Fat: 5g; Carbs: 70g; Protein: 4g; Calcium: 40mg; Sodium: 0mg; Potassium: 250mg; Phosphorus: 50mg

84. Watermelon and Feta Salad

Degree of difficulty: ★☆☆☆☆

Preparation time: 10 mins

Cooking time: 0 mins

Servings: 2

Ingredients:

- 2 teacups cubed watermelon
- 1/2 teacup crumbled feta cheese
- 1/4 teacup fresh mint leaves
- 2 tbsps balsamic reduction

Directions:

1. Organize cubed watermelon on two plates.
2. Spray crumbled feta cheese over the watermelon.
3. Garnish with fresh mint leaves.
4. Spray balsamic reduction over the salad.

Per serving: Calories: 180kcal; Fat: 9g; Carbs: 22g; Protein: 5g; Calcium: 180mg; Sodium: 150mg; Potassium: 300mg; Phosphorus: 100mg

85. Apple and Cranberry Coleslaw

Degree of difficulty: ★★☆☆☆

Preparation time: 15 mins

Cooking time: 0 mins

Servings: 2

Ingredients:

- 2 teacups teared up cabbage
- 1 apple, grated
- 1/4 teacup dried cranberries
- 2 tbsps plain Greek yogurt
- 1 tbsp apple cider vinegar
- 1 tsp honey
- Salt and pepper as required

Directions:

1. Inside a container, blend teared up cabbage, grated apple, and dried cranberries.
2. Inside a distinct container, whisk collectively Greek yogurt, apple cider vinegar, honey, salt, and pepper.
3. Transfer dressing over the coleslaw and shake to cover.

Per serving: Calories: 150kcal; Fat: 1g; Carbs: 35g; Protein: 2g; Calcium: 80mg; Sodium: 30mg; Potassium: 260mg; Phosphorus: 40mg

86. Mackerel and Potato Salad

Degree of difficulty: ★★☆☆☆

Preparation time: 20 mins

Cooking time: 20 mins

Servings: 2

Ingredients:

- 2 mackerel fillets
- 2 teacups cubed boiled potatoes
- 1/2 teacup cubed red onion
- 1/2 teacup cubed celery
- 1/4 teacup plain Greek yogurt
- 2 tbsps fresh dill, severed
- 1 tbsp Dijon mustard
- Salt and pepper as required

Directions:

1. Boil the cubed potatoes till soft, then drain and let them cool.
2. Flavour mackerel fillets with salt and pepper and grill or broil for 4-5 mins on all sides till fully cooked.
3. Inside a big container, blend the cubed potatoes, red onion, celery, plain Greek yogurt, severed dill, Dijon mustard, salt, and pepper.
4. Flake the grilled mackerel and wrap it into the potato salad.
5. Present cold.

Per serving: Calories: 350kcal; Fat: 10g; Carbs: 35g; Protein: 30g; Calcium: 150mg; Sodium: 250mg; Potassium: 600mg; Phosphorus: 500mg

87. Mango and Black Bean Salad

Degree of difficulty: ★☆☆☆☆

Preparation time: 15 mins

Cooking time: 0 mins

Servings: 2

Ingredients:

- 1 ripe mango, cubed
- 1 tin (15 oz) low-sodium black beans, that is drained and washed
- 1/2 teacup cubed red bell pepper
- 1/4 teacup severed fresh cilantro
- 2 tbsps lime juice
- 2 tbsps olive oil
- Salt and pepper as required

Directions:

1. Inside a container, blend cubed mango, black beans, red bell pepper, and fresh cilantro.
2. Inside a small container, whisk collectively your lime juice, olive oil, salt, and pepper.
3. Afterwards, drizzle the dressing across the salad. and shake carefully to blend.

Per serving: Calories: 300kcal; Fat: 10g; Carbs: 47g; Protein: 9g; Calcium: 40mg; Sodium: 10mg; Potassium: 600mg; Phosphorus: 150mg

88. Quinoa and Roasted Vegetable Salad

Degree of difficulty: ★★★☆☆

Preparation time: 20 mins

Cooking time: 30 mins

Servings: 2

Ingredients:

- 1/2 teacup quinoa, washed
- 1 teacup water
- 2 teacups mixed roasted vegetables (e.g., bell peppers, zucchini, and carrots)
- 2 tbsps olive oil
- 2 tbsps balsamic vinegar
- 1 tsp dried thyme
- Salt and pepper as required

Directions:

1. Warm up the oven to 400 deg.F. Shake the mixed vegetables with 1 tbsp of olive oil, dried thyme, salt, and pepper. Roast for 30 mins or 'til soft.
2. Inside your saucepot, boil 1 teacup of water. Include quinoa, decrease temp., cover, then simmer for 15-20 mins till quinoa is cooked and the water is immersed.
3. Inside a big container, blend cooked quinoa and roasted vegetables.
4. Inside a small container, whisk 1 tbsp of olive oil and balsamic vinegar. Afterwards, drizzle the dressing across the salad. and shake to blend.

Per serving: Calories: 320kcal; Fat: 14g; Carbs: 42g; Protein: 8g; Calcium: 50mg; Sodium: 10mg; Potassium: 440mg; Phosphorus: 170mg

89. Cucumber and Dill Salad

Degree of difficulty: ★☆☆☆☆

Preparation time: 10 mins

Cooking time: 0 mins

Servings: 2

Ingredients:

- 2 cucumbers, finely carved
- 1/4 teacup fresh dill, severed
- 1/4 teacup plain Greek yogurt
- 1 tbsp lemon juice
- 1 piece garlic, crushed
- Salt and pepper as required

Directions:

1. Inside a container, blend finely carved cucumbers and severed fresh dill.
2. Inside a distinct container, whisk collectively salt, plain Greek yogurt, lemon juice, crushed garlic, and pepper.
3. Pour the yogurt dressing over the cucumbers and dill. Shake to cover.
4. Present the Cucumber and Dill Salad as a refreshing side dish.

Per serving: Calories: 70kcal; Fat: 1g; Carbs: 12g; Protein: 5g; Calcium: 60mg; Sodium: 20mg; Potassium: 370mg; Phosphorus: 60mg

90. Carrot and Raisin Salad

Degree of difficulty: ★☆☆☆☆

Preparation time: 10 mins

Cooking time: 0 mins

Servings: 2

Ingredients:

- 2 teacups teared up carrots
- 1/4 teacup raisins
- 2 tbsps plain Greek yogurt
- 1 tbsp honey
- 1/2 tsp ground cinnamon

Directions:

1. Inside a container, blend teared up carrots and raisins.
2. Inside a distinct container, whisk collectively plain Greek yogurt, honey, and ground cinnamon.
3. Pour the yogurt dressing over the carrot and raisin solution. Shake to cover.
4. Present the Carrot and Raisin Salad as a sweet and crunchy side dish.

Per serving: Calories: 120kcal; Fat: 1g; Carbs: 29g; Protein: 2g; Calcium: 60mg; Sodium: 40mg; Potassium: 370mg; Phosphorus: 50mg

91. Beetroot and Orange Salad

Degree of difficulty: ★★☆☆☆

Preparation time: 15 mins

Cooking time: 0 mins

Servings: 2

Ingredients:

- 2 medium beetroots, cooked, skinned, and cubed
- 2 oranges, skinned and segmented
- 1/4 teacup severed fresh parsley
- 1/4 teacup severed walnuts

For Lemon Vinaigrette:

- Juice and zest of 1 lemon
- 2 tbsps olive oil
- 1 tsp Dijon mustard
- Salt and pepper as required

Directions:

1. Inside a container, blend cubed cooked beetroots, orange segments, severed fresh parsley, and severed walnuts.
2. Inside a mini container, whisk collectively lemon juice, lemon zest, olive oil, Dijon mustard, salt, and pepper to make the vinaigrette.
3. Spray the lemon vinaigrette over the salad then shake to cover.
4. Present the Beetroot and Orange Salad for a colorful and flavorful side dish.

Per serving: Calories: 180kcal; Fat: 7g; Carbs: 28g; Protein: 4g; Calcium: 90mg; Sodium: 70mg; Potassium: 570mg; Phosphorus: 70mg

Kidney-Friendly Snacks

92. Carrot Sticks with Hummus

Degree of difficulty: ★☆☆☆☆

Preparation time: 5 mins

Cooking time: 0 mins

Servings: 2

Ingredients:

- 2 medium-sized carrots, skinned and cut into sticks
- 4 tbsps of low-sodium hummus

Directions:

1. Wash, skin, then cut the carrots into sticks.
2. Present the carrot sticks with the low-sodium hummus for dipping.

Per serving: Calories: 75kcal; Fat: 4g; Carbs: 8g; Protein: 2g; Calcium: 38mg; Sodium: 80mg; Potassium: 210mg; Phosphorus: 50mg

93. Celery and Peanut Butter

Degree of difficulty: ★☆☆☆☆

Preparation time: 5 mins

Cooking time: 0 mins

Servings: 2

Ingredients:

- 4 celery stalks, cut into manageable pieces
- 2 tbsps of unsweetened peanut butter

Directions:

1. Wash and cut the celery into manageable pieces.
2. Disperse a small amount of unsweetened peanut butter on the celery pieces.

Per serving: Calories: 90kcal; Fat: 7g; Carbs: 4g; Protein: 3g; Calcium: 40mg; Sodium: 60mg; Potassium: 250mg; Phosphorus: 60mg

94. Hard-Boiled Eggs Degree of difficulty: ★★☆☆☆

Preparation time: 5 mins

Cooking time: 10 mins

Servings: 2

Ingredients:

- 4 big eggs
- Water for boiling

Directions:

1. Place eggs in saucepot then include sufficient water to cover them.
2. Boil the water, then decrease the temp. then simmer for 10 mins.
3. Take out the eggs from the heat and put them in cold water to cool.
4. Once cooled, peel the eggs and present.

Per serving: Calories: 140kcal; Fat: 10g; Carbs: 1g; Protein: 12g; Calcium: 56mg; Sodium: 126mg; Potassium: 130mg; Phosphorus: 96mg

95. Fresh Fruit Salad

Degree of difficulty: ★☆☆☆☆

Preparation time: 10 mins

Cooking time: 0 mins

Servings: 2

Ingredients:

- 1 teacup of mixed fresh fruit (e.g., melon, berries, grapes)
- 1 tbsp of fresh lime or your lemon juice
- Fresh mint leaves for garnish (elective)

Directions:

1. Wash and prepare the mixed fresh fruit, cutting them into bite-sized pieces if necessary.
2. Shake the fruit with fresh lime or lemon juice.
3. Garnish with fresh mint leaves if anticipated.

Per serving: Calories: 60kcal; Fat: 0g; Carbs: 16g; Protein: 1g; Calcium: 10mg; Sodium: 0mg; Potassium: 150mg; Phosphorus: 10mg

96. Watermelon Cubes

Degree of difficulty: ★☆☆☆☆

Preparation time: 5 mins

Cooking time: 0 mins

Servings: 2

Ingredients:

- 2 teacups of watermelon, cubed

Directions:

1. Wash and cube the watermelon.
2. Present the watermelon cubes inside a container.

Per serving: Calories: 30kcal; Fat: 0g; Carbs: 8g; Protein: 1g; Calcium: 10mg; Sodium: 0mg; Potassium: 120mg; Phosphorus: 10mg

97. Sliced Cucumber with Lemon

Degree of difficulty: ★☆☆☆☆

Preparation time: 5 mins

Cooking time: 0 mins

Servings: 2

Ingredients:

- 1 cucumber, finely carved
- 1 lemon, juiced
- Fresh dill or parsley for garnish (elective)

Directions:

1. Wash and slice the cucumber.
2. Spray lemon juice over the cucumber slices.
3. Garnish using fresh dill or parsley if anticipated.

Per serving: Calories: 15kcal; Fat: 0g; Carbs: 4g; Protein: 1g; Calcium: 20mg; Sodium: 0mg; Potassium: 200mg; Phosphorus: 20mg

98. Berries with Whipped Cream

Degree of difficulty: ★★☆☆☆

Preparation time: 5 mins

Cooking time: 0 mins

Servings: 2

Ingredients:

- 1 teacup of mixed berries (e.g., strawberries, blueberries, raspberries)
- 1/2 teacup of unsweetened whipped cream

Directions:

1. Wash the mixed berries and put them in serving containers.
2. Top every container with a dollop of unsweetened whipped cream.

Per serving: Calories: 100kcal; Fat: 8g; Carbs: 8g; Protein: 1g; Calcium: 20mg; Sodium: 0mg; Potassium: 100mg; Phosphorus: 20mg

99. Edamame

Degree of difficulty: ★★☆☆☆

Preparation time: 5 mins

Cooking time: 5 mins

Servings: 2

Ingredients:

- 1 teacup of frozen shelled edamame
- 1/2 tsp of low-sodium soy sauce (elective)

Directions:

1. Boil edamame in your salted water for 5 mins, or 'til soft.
2. Drain and, if anticipated, shake with a small amount of low-sodium soy sauce.

Per serving: Calories: 90kcal; Fat: 3g; Carbs: 8g; Protein: 8g; Calcium: 50mg; Sodium: 10mg; Potassium: 220mg; Phosphorus: 100mg

100.   Greek Yogurt with Honey

Degree of difficulty: ★☆☆☆☆

Preparation time: 5 mins

Cooking time: 0 mins

Servings: 2

Ingredients:

- 1 teacup of low-fat Greek yogurt
- 2 tbsps of honey

Directions:

1. Split the Greek yogurt evenly among two containers.
2. Spray 1 tbsp of honey over each serving of yogurt.
3. Mix the honey into yogurt and relish.

Per serving: Calories: 170kcal; Fat: 0g; Carbs: 35g; Protein: 10g; Calcium: 200mg; Sodium: 60mg; Potassium: 200mg; Phosphorus: 140mg

101.   Pita Bread with Hummus

Degree of difficulty: ★★☆☆☆

Preparation time: 5 mins

Cooking time: 0 mins

Servings: 2

Ingredients:

- 2 wheat pita bread rounds
- 4 tbsps of low-sodium hummus

Directions:

1. Cut each wheat pita bread round into halves or quarters.
2. Warm the pita bread briefly if anticipated.
3. Present with low-sodium hummus for dipping.

Per serving: Calories: 180kcal; Fat: 4g; Carbs: 32g; Protein: 6g; Calcium: 40mg; Sodium: 80mg; Potassium: 100mg; Phosphorus: 100mg

102.   Dried Apricots

Degree of difficulty: ★☆☆☆☆

Preparation time: 2 mins

Cooking time: 0 mins

Servings: 2

Ingredients:

- 8 dried apricots

Directions:

1. Measure out 8 dried apricots.
2. Relish the dried apricots as a sweet and nourishing snack.

Per serving: Calories: 80kcal; Fat: 0g; Carbs: 20g; Protein: 1g; Calcium: 20mg; Sodium: 5mg; Potassium: 420mg; Phosphorus: 20mg

103.   Cheese and Whole Wheat Crackers

Degree of difficulty: ★☆☆☆☆

Preparation time: 2 mins

Cooking time: 0 mins

Servings: 2

Ingredients:

- 2 oz. of low-sodium cheese (e.g., Swiss or cheddar)
- 6 whole wheat crackers

Directions:

1. Cut the low-sodium cheese into bite-sized pieces.
2. Present the cheese with whole wheat crackers.

Per serving: Calories: 180kcal; Fat: 10g; Carbs: 15g; Protein: 10g; Calcium: 200mg; Sodium: 50mg; Potassium: 60mg; Phosphorus: 150mg

104.   *Popcorn*

Degree of difficulty: ★☆☆☆☆

Preparation time: 5 mins

Cooking time: 3 mins

Servings: 2

Ingredients:

- 1/4 teacup of low-sodium popcorn kernels
- 1 tbsp of olive oil (for popping)
- Seasoning (elective): A tweak of herbs or spices like thyme or rosemary

Directions:

1. Place popcorn kernels in microwave-safe container and spray with olive oil. Include elective seasoning.
2. Cover container using a microwave-safe plate and microwave on high for 3 mins or 'til the popping slows down to 2 secs among pops.
3. Carefully take out container from the microwave and allow it to cool prior to presenting.

Per serving: Calories: 75kcal; Fat: 4g; Carbs: 8g; Protein: 1g; Calcium: 0mg; Sodium: 0mg; Potassium: 35mg; Phosphorus: 35mg

105.   *Baked Sweet Potato Fries*

Degree of difficulty: ★★★☆☆

Preparation time: 10 mins

Cooking time: 25 mins

Servings: 2

Ingredients:

- 2 small sweet potatoes, cut into fries
- 1 tbsp of olive oil
- Seasoning (e.g., paprika, garlic powder, or rosemary) (elective)

Directions:

1. Warm up the oven to 425 deg.F.
2. Shake sweet potato fries using olive oil and any desired seasonings.
3. Disperse the fries on a baking sheet then bake for 25 mins, turning them halfway through, or 'til they're crispy on the outside and soft on the inside.

Per serving: Calories: 150kcal; Fat: 6g; Carbs: 23g; Protein: 2g; Calcium: 30mg; Sodium: 20mg; Potassium: 380mg; Phosphorus: 60mg

106.   *Cottage Cheese and Sliced Peaches*

Degree of difficulty: ★☆☆☆☆

Preparation time: 5 mins

Cooking time: 0 mins

Servings: 2

Ingredients:

- 1 teacup of low-fat cottage cheese
- 1 fresh peach, carved

Directions:

1. Spoon half a teacup of low-fat cottage cheese into each serving container.
2. Top with carved fresh peaches and relish.

Per serving: Calories: 160kcal; Fat: 2g; Carbs: 18g; Protein: 18g; Calcium: 140mg; Sodium: 330mg; Potassium: 260mg; Phosphorus: 270mg

107.   *Rice Cakes with Almond Butter*

Degree of difficulty: ★☆☆☆☆

Preparation time: 2 mins

Cooking time: 0 mins

Servings: 2

Ingredients:

- 4 rice cakes
- 4 tbsps of unsalted almond butter

Directions:

1. Disperse 1 tbsp of your almond butter on each rice cake.
2. Present and relish as a snack.

Per serving: Calories: 190kcal; Fat: 12g; Carbs: 15g; Protein: 5g; Calcium: 80mg; Sodium: 0mg; Potassium: 100mg; Phosphorus: 100mg

108.   *Fig and Walnut Bites*

Degree of difficulty: ★★☆☆☆

Preparation time: 10 mins

Cooking time: 0 mins

Servings: 2

Ingredients:

- 4 dried figs, quartered
- 1/4 teacup of walnuts, severed

Directions:

1. Organize the quartered dried figs and severed walnuts on a plate.
2. Relish these as a delightful and quick snack.

Per serving: Calories: 160kcal; Fat: 8g; Carbs: 22g; Protein: 3g; Calcium: 60mg; Sodium: 0mg; Potassium: 280mg; Phosphorus: 80mg

109.   *Sliced Bell Peppers*

Degree of difficulty: ★☆☆☆☆

Preparation time: 5 mins

Cooking time: 0 mins

Servings: 2

Ingredients:

- 1 red bell pepper, carved
- 1 green bell pepper, carved

Directions:

1. Wash and slice the red and green bell peppers into strips.
2. Organize bell pepper slices on a plate for a crunchy and colorful snack.

Per serving: Calories: 30kcal; Fat: 0g; Carbs: 7g; Protein: 1g; Calcium: 10mg; Sodium: 5mg; Potassium: 190mg; Phosphorus: 20mg

110.   *Baked Apple Chips*

Degree of difficulty: ★☆☆☆☆

Preparation time: 10 mins

Cooking time: 2 hrs

Servings: 2

Ingredients:

- 2 apples, finely carved (use a mandoline slicer for uniform slices)
- 1/2 tsp ground cinnamon (elective)
- Cooking spray

Directions:

1. Warm up your oven to 200 deg.F.
2. Put the finely carved apples on a baking sheet covered with parchment paper.
3. If anticipated, spray the apple slices with ground cinnamon.
4. Bake into your warmed up oven for 2 hrs or 'til the apple slices are crisp and mildly golden.
5. Allow the Baked Apple Chips to cool prior to presenting.

Per serving: Calories: 60kcal; Fat: 0g; Carbs: 16g; Protein: 0g; Calcium: 10mg; Sodium: 0mg; Potassium: 130mg; Phosphorus: 10mg

111. Carrot and Celery Sticks with Hummus

Degree of difficulty: ★☆☆☆☆

Preparation time: 10 mins

Cooking time: 0 mins

Servings: 2

Ingredients:

- 2 carrots, skinned and cut into sticks
- 2 celery stalks, cut into sticks
- 1/2 teacup renal-friendly hummus (store-bought or homemade)

Directions:

1. Organize the carrot and celery sticks on a plate.
2. Present them with renal-friendly hummus for dipping.
3. Relish this healthy and crunchy snack!

Per serving: Calories: 100kcal; Fat: 4g; Carbs: 14g; Protein: 4g; Calcium: 60mg; Sodium: 200mg; Potassium: 310mg; Phosphorus: 70mg

112.   Baked Zucchini Chips

Degree of difficulty: ★★☆☆☆

Preparation time: 15 mins

Cooking time: 25 mins

Servings: 2

Ingredients:

- 2 small zucchinis, finely carved
- 1/4 teacup grated Parmesan cheese
- 1/2 tsp garlic powder
- Salt and pepper as required
- Cooking spray

Directions:

1. Warm up oven to 425 deg.F then line your baking sheet using parchment paper.
2. Inside a container, blend finely carved zucchinis, grated Parmesan cheese, garlic powder, salt, and pepper. Shake to cover the zucchini slices.
3. Organize the covered zucchini slices on the prepared baking sheet.
4. Mildly spray the zucchini slices with cooking spray.
5. Bake into your warmed up oven for 20-25 mins or 'til the zucchini chips are crisp and golden.
6. Allow the Baked Zucchini Chips to cool prior to presenting.

Per serving: Calories: 70kcal; Fat: 3g; Carbs: 6g; Protein: 5g; Calcium: 90mg; Sodium: 220mg; Potassium: 400mg; Phosphorus: 70mg

Appetizers and Tasty Side Dishes

113.   Asparagus Wrapped in Turkey

Degree of difficulty: ★★☆☆☆

Preparation time: 10 mins

Cooking time: 15 mins

Servings: 2

Ingredients:

- 12 asparagus spears, clipped
- 4 slices low-sodium turkey breast
- Olive oil for brushing
- Salt and pepper as required

Directions:

1. Warm up your oven to 400 deg.F.
2. Shake asparagus using a little olive oil, salt, and pepper.
3. Bundle 3 asparagus spears together and wrap each bundle with a slice of turkey.
4. Place bundles on a baking sheet and roast for 15 mins or 'til the asparagus is soft and the turkey is mildly crispy.

Per serving: Calories: 80kcal; Fat: 1g; Carbs: 4g; Protein: 14g; Calcium: 30mg; Sodium: 180mg; Potassium: 200mg; Phosphorus: 50mg

114.   Broccoli and Walnut Salad

Degree of difficulty: ★★☆☆☆

Preparation time: 10 mins

Cooking time: 5 mins

Servings: 2

Ingredients:

- 4 teacups fresh broccoli florets, blanched and cooled
- 1/4 teacup severed walnuts
- 2 tbsps olive oil
- 1 tbsp lemon juice
- 1 piece garlic, crushed
- Salt and pepper as required

Directions:

1. Inside a big container, blend the blanched broccoli florets and severed walnuts.
2. Inside a distinct container, whisk collectively the salt, olive oil, lemon juice, crushed garlic, and pepper.
3. Afterwards, drizzle the dressing across the salad. and shake to blend.

Per serving: Calories: 210kcal; Fat: 18g; Carbs: 9g; Protein: 5g; Calcium: 60mg; Sodium: 30mg; Potassium: 400mg; Phosphorus: 90mg

115.   Roasted Eggplant Dip

Degree of difficulty: ★★☆☆☆

Preparation time: 15 mins

Cooking time: 30 mins

Servings: 2

Ingredients:

- 1 medium eggplant
- 2 pieces garlic, crushed
- 2 tbsps olive oil
- 1 tbsp lemon juice
- Salt and pepper as required

Directions:

1. Warm up your oven to 400 deg.F.
2. Cut the eggplant in half and place it, cut side down, on a baking sheet. Roast for 30 mins 'til the flesh is soft.
3. Let eggplant to cool, then scoop out the flesh into a container.
4. Mash the roasted eggplant and mix with crushed garlic, olive oil, and lemon juice. Flavour with salt and pepper.

Per serving: Calories: 150kcal; Fat: 14g; Carbs: 6g; Protein: 2g; Calcium: 20mg; Sodium: 10mg; Potassium: 250mg; Phosphorus: 40mg

116. Rice Pilaf with Mixed Veggies

Degree of difficulty: ★★★☆☆
Preparation time: 10 mins
Cooking time: 25 mins
Servings: 2
Ingredients:

- 1/2 teacup long-grain white rice
- 1 teacup low-sodium chicken or vegetable broth
- 1/2 teacup mixed vegetables (peas, carrots, corn)
- 1/4 tsp dried thyme
- Salt and pepper as required

Directions:

1. Inside your saucepot, blend the rice and broth. Boil, then decrease temp. to low, cover, then simmer for 15 mins.
2. Include mixed vegetables and dried thyme to the rice. Continue to cook for an extra 10 mins or 'til the rice is soft and the liquid is immersed.
3. Flavour with salt and pepper.

Per serving: Calories: 180kcal; Fat: 1g; Carbs: 40g; Protein: 4g; Calcium: 20mg; Sodium: 60mg; Potassium: 150mg; Phosphorus: 100mg

117. Deviled Eggs

Degree of difficulty: ★★☆☆☆
Preparation time: 15 mins
Cooking time: 10 mins
Servings: 2
Ingredients:

- 2 hard-boiled eggs
- 1 tbsp mayonnaise
- 1/2 tsp Dijon mustard
- Paprika for garnish (elective)

Directions:

1. Slice hard-boiled eggs in half then take out the yolks.
2. Inside a container, mash the egg yolks with mayonnaise and Dijon mustard.
3. Spoon your yolk solution back into egg white halves.
4. Spray with paprika if anticipated.

Per serving: Calories: 120kcal; Fat: 9g; Carbs: 1g; Protein: 7g; Calcium: 30mg; Sodium: 60mg; Potassium: 80mg; Phosphorus: 100mg

118. Greek Potato Salad

Degree of difficulty: ★★☆☆☆
Preparation time: 15 mins
Cooking time: 20 mins
Servings: 2
Ingredients:

- 2 teacups boiled and cubed red potatoes
- 1/4 teacup severed cucumber
- 1/4 teacup severed red onion
- 1/4 teacup Kalamata olives, that is eroded and carved
- 2 tbsps crumbled feta cheese
- 2 tbsps olive oil
- 1 tbsp lemon juice
- 1/2 tsp dried oregano
- Salt and pepper as required

Directions:

1. Inside a container, blend the Kalamata olives, cubed red potatoes, severed cucumber, red onion, and crumbled feta cheese.
2. Inside a distinct container, whisk collectively your olive oil, lemon juice, dried oregano, salt, and pepper.
3. Afterwards, drizzle the dressing across the salad. and shake to blend.

Per serving: Calories: 320kcal; Fat: 20g; Carbs: 30g; Protein: 5g; Calcium: 90mg; Sodium: 370mg; Potassium: 500mg; Phosphorus: 90mg

119. **Caprese Quinoa Salad**

Degree of difficulty: ★★☆☆☆

Preparation time: 15 mins

Cooking time: 15 mins

Servings: 2

Ingredients:

- 1 teacup cooked quinoa, cooled
- 1 teacup cherry tomatoes, divided
- 1/2 teacup fresh basil leaves, torn
- 1/2 teacup fresh mozzarella balls (bocconcini)
- Balsamic glaze for drizzling (elective)

Directions:

1. Inside a container, blend the cooked quinoa, cherry tomatoes, torn basil leaves, and mozzarella balls.
2. Spray with balsamic glaze if anticipated.

Per serving: Calories: 320kcal; Fat: 12g; Carbs: 35g; Protein: 15g; Calcium: 150mg; Sodium: 60mg; Potassium: 400mg; Phosphorus: 200mg

120. **Spinach and Feta Stuffed Mushrooms**

Degree of difficulty: ★★★☆☆

Preparation time: 15 mins

Cooking time: 20 mins

Servings: 2

Ingredients:

- 4 big mushrooms, that is stems taken out and finely severed
- 1 teacup fresh spinach, severed
- 1/4 teacup crumbled feta cheese
- 2 pieces garlic, crushed
- Salt and pepper as required

Directions:

1. Warm up your oven to 350 deg.F.
2. In griddle, sauté the mushroom stems, severed spinach, and crushed garlic till softened.
3. Flavour with salt and pepper.
4. Fill the mushroom caps with the sautéed solution and top with crumbled feta cheese.
5. Place filled mushrooms in a baking dish then bake for 20 mins till soft.

Per serving: Calories: 90kcal; Fat: 6g; Carbs: 6g; Protein: 5g; Calcium: 80mg; Sodium: 230mg; Potassium: 400mg; Phosphorus: 80mg

121. **Baked Artichoke Hearts**

Degree of difficulty: ★★☆☆☆

Preparation time: 10 mins

Cooking time: 25 mins

Servings: 2

Ingredients:

- 1 tin (14 oz) of artichoke hearts, drained and divided
- 2 tbsps olive oil
- 2 pieces garlic, crushed
- 1/4 teacup grated Parmesan cheese (elective)
- Salt and pepper as required

Directions:

1. Warm up your oven to 375 deg.F.
2. In baking dish, place the divided artichoke hearts.
3. Spray with olive oil, then spray crushed garlic, salt, and pepper over the artichokes.
4. If anticipated, top with grated Parmesan cheese.
5. Bake for 25 mins or 'til the artichoke hearts are soft and mildly browned.

Per serving: Calories: 180kcal; Fat: 14g; Carbs: 8g; Protein: 5g; Calcium: 150mg; Sodium: 360mg; Potassium: 190mg; Phosphorus: 100mg

122. Guacamole with Veggie Sticks

Degree of difficulty: ★★☆☆☆

Preparation time: 10 mins

Cooking time: 0 mins

Servings: 2

Ingredients:

- 1 ripe avocado, mashed
- 1 small tomato, cubed
- 1/4 teacup red onion, finely severed
- 1 piece garlic, crushed
- 1 tbsp fresh lime juice
- Salt and pepper as required
- Carrot and cucumber sticks for dipping

Directions:

1. Inside a container, blend the mashed avocado, cubed tomato, severed red onion, crushed garlic, and fresh lime juice.
2. Blend thoroughly then flavour using salt and pepper as required.
3. Present the guacamole with carrot and cucumber sticks for dipping.

Per serving: Calories: 150kcal; Fat: 12g; Carbs: 10g; Protein: 2g; Calcium: 20mg; Sodium: 5mg; Potassium: 370mg; Phosphorus: 60mg

123. Lemon-Dill Cucumber Salad

Degree of difficulty: ★☆☆☆☆

Preparation time: 10 mins

Cooking time: 0 mins

Servings: 2

Ingredients:

- 1 cucumber, finely carved
- 1 tbsp fresh dill, severed
- 2 tbsps lemon juice
- 1 tbsp olive oil
- Salt and pepper as required

Directions:

1. Inside a container, blend the finely carved cucumber, severed dill, lemon juice, and olive oil.
2. Flavour with salt and pepper as required.
3. Shake everything together and present.

Per serving: Calories: 70kcal; Fat: 5g; Carbs: 6g; Protein: 1g; Calcium: 20mg; Sodium: 10mg; Potassium: 250mg; Phosphorus: 20mg

124. Mashed Cauliflower

Degree of difficulty: ★★☆☆☆

Preparation time: 10 mins

Cooking time: 15 mins

Servings: 2

Ingredients:

- 1 small head of cauliflower, that is cut into florets
- 1 piece garlic, crushed
- 2 tbsps low-fat cream cheese (elective)
- Salt and pepper as required

Directions:

1. Steam or boil cauliflower florets till soft.
2. Drain cauliflower then transfer it to a container.
3. Mash the cauliflower, adding crushed garlic, and low-fat cream cheese (if anticipated) for creaminess.
4. Flavour with salt and pepper.

Per serving: Calories: 60kcal; Fat: 2g; Carbs: 9g; Protein: 3g; Calcium: 40mg; Sodium: 60mg; Potassium: 440mg; Phosphorus: 70mg

125. *Caprese Skewers*

Degree of difficulty: ★☆☆☆☆

Preparation time: 10 mins

Cooking time: 0 mins

Servings: 2

Ingredients:

- 12 cherry tomatoes
- 12 fresh basil leaves
- 12 small mozzarella balls (bocconcini)
- Balsamic glaze for drizzling (elective)

Directions:

1. Thread a cherry tomato, basil leaf, and mozzarella ball onto each skewer.
2. Spray with balsamic glaze if anticipated.

Per serving: Calories: 150kcal; Fat: 8g; Carbs: 4g; Protein: 10g; Calcium: 250mg; Sodium: 50mg; Potassium: 150mg; Phosphorus: 100mg

126. *Roasted Brussels Sprouts*

Degree of difficulty: ★★☆☆☆

Preparation time: 10 mins

Cooking time: 25 mins

Servings: 2

Ingredients:

- 2 teacups Brussels sprouts, clipped and divided
- 2 tbsps olive oil
- Salt and pepper as required

Directions:

1. Warm up your oven to 400 deg.F.
2. Shake the Brussels sprouts using olive oil, salt, and pepper.
3. Disperse them on your baking sheet in a single layer.
4. Roast for 25 mins 'til they are soft and mildly browned.

Per serving: Calories: 100kcal; Fat: 7g; Carbs: 9g; Protein: 3g; Calcium: 40mg; Sodium: 25mg; Potassium: 450mg; Phosphorus: 70mg

127. *Green Bean Almondine*

Degree of difficulty: ★★☆☆☆

Preparation time: 10 mins

Cooking time: 10 mins

Servings: 2

Ingredients:

- 2 teacups fresh green beans, clipped
- 2 tbsps carved almonds
- 1 tbsp olive oil
- 1 tbsp fresh lemon juice
- Salt and pepper as required

Directions:

1. Steam green beans till they are soft-crisp, around 5-7 mins.
2. In griddle, warm the olive oil and toast the carved almonds till they are golden brown.
3. Shake the steamed green beans with the toasted almonds, lemon juice, salt, and pepper.

Per serving: Calories: 110kcal; Fat: 8g; Carbs: 8g; Protein: 3g; Calcium: 40mg; Sodium: 10mg; Potassium: 280mg; Phosphorus: 60mg

128. Roasted Garlic Cauliflower

Degree of difficulty: ★★☆☆☆

Preparation time: 10 mins

Cooking time: 25 mins

Servings: 2

Ingredients:

- 1 small head of cauliflower, that is cut into florets
- 2 pieces garlic, crushed
- 1 tbsp olive oil
- 1/2 tsp dried thyme
- Salt and pepper as required
- Fresh parsley for garnish (elective)

Directions:

1. Warm up your oven to 425 deg.F.
2. Inside a big container, blend cauliflower florets, salt, crushed garlic, olive oil, dried thyme, and pepper. Shake to cover the cauliflower.
3. Disperse the covered cauliflower on your baking sheet.
4. Roast into your warmed up oven for 20-25 mins or 'til the cauliflower is soft and mildly browned.
5. Garnish with fresh parsley prior to presenting.

Per serving: Calories: 70kcal; Fat: 4g; Carbs: 8g; Protein: 3g; Calcium: 30mg; Sodium: 35mg; Potassium: 410mg; Phosphorus: 60mg

129. Steamed Asparagus with Lemon

Degree of difficulty: ★☆☆☆☆

Preparation time: 10 mins

Cooking time: 5 mins

Servings: 2

Ingredients:

- 1 bunch of fresh asparagus, clipped
- 1 lemon, finely carved
- 1 tbsp olive oil
- Salt and pepper as required

Directions:

1. Steam the clipped asparagus till soft, about 3-5 mins.
2. In your griddle, warm olive oil in a middling temp. Include lemon slices and cook for a min till they start to caramelize.
3. Organize the steamed asparagus on a plate, top with caramelized lemon slices, and flavour using salt and pepper.
4. Present the Steamed Asparagus with Lemon as a delightful side dish.

Per serving: Calories: 50kcal; Fat: 4g; Carbs: 4g; Protein: 2g; Calcium: 30mg; Sodium: 0mg; Potassium: 270mg; Phosphorus: 50mg

130. Cucumber and Mint Yogurt Dip

Degree of difficulty: ★☆☆☆☆

Preparation time: 10 mins

Cooking time: 0 mins

Servings: 2

Ingredients:

- 1 cucumber, finely grated and drained
- 1 teacup plain Greek yogurt
- 2 tbsps fresh mint leaves, severed
- 1 piece garlic, crushed
- Salt and pepper as required

Directions:

1. Inside a container, blend finely grated and drained cucumber, plain Greek yogurt, severed fresh mint leaves, crushed garlic, salt, and pepper. Blend thoroughly.
2. Put in the fridge the Cucumber and Mint Yogurt Dip for 30 mins to let the flavors to meld.
3. Present the dip with fresh vegetables or whole-grain crackers.

Per serving: Calories: 90kcal; Fat: 1g; Carbs: 8g; Protein: 12g; Calcium: 120mg; Sodium: 40mg; Potassium: 340mg; Phosphorus: 80mg

Dessert

131.   *Poached Pears in Red Wine*

Degree of difficulty: ★★☆☆☆

Preparation time: 10 mins

Cooking time: 20 mins

Servings: 2

Ingredients:

- 2 ripe pears, skinned and cored
- 1 teacup red wine
- 1/2 teacup water
- 2 tbsps honey
- 1 cinnamon stick
- 1 strip of orange zest (elective)

Directions:

1. Inside your saucepot, blend the red wine, water, honey, cinnamon stick, and elective orange zest.
2. Bring the solution to a simmer.
3. Include skinned and cored pears to the simmering liquid.
4. Simmer for 15-20 mins or 'til the pears are soft but not mushy. Turn them occasionally to ensure even cooking.
5. Take out pears and allow the poaching liquid to reduce if anticipated.
6. Present the pears with a spray of the reduced poaching liquid.

Per serving: Calories: 180kcal; Fat: 0g; Carbs: 40g; Protein: 1g; Calcium: 10mg; Sodium: 5mg; Potassium: 200mg; Phosphorus: 20mg

132.   *Fig and Ricotta Bruschetta*

Degree of difficulty: ★★☆☆☆

Preparation time: 15 mins

Cooking time: 5 mins

Servings: 2

Ingredients:

- 4 fresh figs, divided
- 4 slices of grain bread
- 1/2 teacup low-fat ricotta cheese
- 1 tbsp honey
- A tweak of cinnamon (elective)

Directions:

1. Warm up your grill or oven in a med-high temp.
2. Grill or toast the grain bread till it's crispy and golden brown.
3. Inside a container, mix the low-fat ricotta cheese with honey and elective cinnamon.
4. Place divided figs on the grill or under the broiler for 2-3 mins on all sides till they caramelize mildly.
5. Disperse the sweetened ricotta solution on the toasted bread slices.
6. Top each slice with grilled fig halves.
7. Present your fig and ricotta bruschetta.

Per serving: Calories: 250kcal; Fat: 5g; Carbs: 48g; Protein: 7g; Calcium: 180mg; Sodium: 210mg; Potassium: 250mg; Phosphorus: 140mg

133. **Berry Parfait with Whipped Cream**

Degree of difficulty: ★☆☆☆☆

Preparation time: 10 mins

Cooking time: 0 mins

Servings: 2

Ingredients:

- 1 teacup mixed berries (e.g., strawberries, blueberries, raspberries)
- 1/2 teacup low-fat whipped cream
- 1/4 teacup low-sugar granola
- 1/2 tsp honey

Directions:

1. Wash and prepare the berries.
2. In two serving glasses or containers, layer half of the berries at the bottom.
3. Place a dollop of whipped cream on top of the berries.
4. Spray a portion of granola over the whipped cream.
5. Replicate the layering with the remaining berries, whipped cream, and granola.
6. Spray a little honey on top if anticipated (keep it minimal for low sugar).
7. Present instantly.

Per serving: Calories: 150kcal; Fat: 5g; Carbs: 25g; Protein: 2g; Calcium: 40mg; Sodium: 10mg; Potassium: 150mg; Phosphorus: 50mg

134. **Pumpkin Custard**

Degree of difficulty: ★★★☆☆

Preparation time: 15 mins

Cooking time: 30 mins

Servings: 2

Ingredients:

- 1 teacup tinned pumpkin puree (unsweetened)
- 1/2 teacup low-fat milk
- 1/4 teacup honey
- 1/2 tsp ground cinnamon
- 1/4 tsp ground nutmeg
- 1/4 tsp vanilla extract
- 2 eggs

Directions:

1. Warm up your oven to 350 deg.F.
2. Inside a blending container, blend the pumpkin puree, low-fat milk, honey, ground cinnamon, ground nutmeg, and vanilla extract.
3. Inside a distinct container, beat the eggs then stir them into the pumpkin solution.
4. Pour custard into two ramekins.
5. Place ramekins in baking dish then include hot water to the dish to create a water bath.
6. Bake for 30 mins or 'til the custard is set but still mildly jiggly in the center.
7. Allow it to cool and then put in the fridge prior to presenting.

Per serving: Calories: 220kcal; Fat: 6g; Carbs: 35g; Protein: 8g; Calcium: 170mg; Sodium: 70mg; Potassium: 270mg; Phosphorus: 120mg

135. *Pomegranate Granita*

Degree of difficulty: ★★☆☆☆

Preparation time: 15 mins

Cooking time: 0 mins

Servings: 2

Ingredients:

- 1 teacup pomegranate juice (unsweetened)
- 2 tbsps honey
- 1 tbsp fresh lemon juice

Directions:

1. Inside a container, blend the pomegranate juice, honey, and fresh lemon juice. Blend thoroughly till the sweetener is dissolved.
2. Pour solution into a shallow dish.
3. Place dish in the freezer and allow it to freeze for 30 mins.
4. Use fork to scrape the partially frozen solution to form granules.
5. Return the dish to the freezer and repeat the scraping process every 30 mins for a total of 3-4 hrs.
6. Once you have a fluffy, granita-like texture, present in chilled containers.

Per serving: Calories: 120kcal; Fat: 0g; Carbs: 31g; Protein: 0g; Calcium: 10mg; Sodium: 5mg; Potassium: 250mg; Phosphorus: 10mg

136. *Mixed Berry Compote*

Degree of difficulty: ★★☆☆☆

Preparation time: 10 mins

Cooking time: 10 mins

Servings: 2

Ingredients:

- 1 teacup mixed berries (strawberries, blueberries, raspberries)
- 2 tbsps honey
- 1/4 tsp vanilla extract
- 1/4 teacup water
- Zest of one lemon (elective)

Directions:

1. Inside your saucepot, blend the mixed berries, honey, vanilla extract, and water.
2. If anticipated, include lemon zest for extra flavor.
3. Cook in a low heat, mixing irregularly, for 10 mins or 'til the berries soften and the solution thickens.
4. Allow the compote to cool.
5. Present the mixed berry compote as a topping for low-potassium pancakes or desserts.

Per serving: Calories: 80kcal; Fat: 0g; Carbs: 21g; Protein: 1g; Calcium: 10mg; Sodium: 0mg; Potassium: 90mg; Phosphorus: 10mg

137. Baked Apple with Cinnamon

Degree of difficulty: ★☆☆☆☆

Preparation time: 10 mins

Cooking time: 30 mins

Servings: 2

Ingredients:

- 2 medium-sized apples
- 1/2 tsp ground cinnamon
- 1/4 tsp ground nutmeg
- 1 tbsp brown sugar (elective, for sweetness)

Directions:

1. Warm up your oven to 350 deg.F.
2. Wash and core the apples, removing the seeds and a bit of flesh to create a well in the center.
3. Place apples in an oven-safe dish.
4. Spray cinnamon and nutmeg inside the cored apples.
5. If anticipated, spray a bit of brown sugar into each apple for sweetness.
6. Cover the dish using foil then bake for 30 mins, or 'til the apples are soft.
7. Present the baked apples warm.

Per serving: Calories: 90kcal; Fat: 0.5g; Carbs: 24g; Protein: 0.5g; Calcium: 10mg; Sodium: 0mg; Potassium: 190mg; Phosphorus: 10mg

138. Peach Sorbet

Degree of difficulty: ★★☆☆☆

Preparation time: 10 mins

Cooking time: 0 mins

Servings: 2

Ingredients:

- 2 ripe peaches, skinned and eroded
- 2 tbsps honey
- 1/2 teacup ice cubes
- 1/2 teacup water

Directions:

1. In mixer, blend the skinned and eroded peaches, honey, ice cubes, and water.
2. Blend till smooth.
3. If the sorbet is too thick, you can include a little more water.
4. Pour sorbet into serving dishes.
5. Present instantly.

Per serving: Calories: 120kcal; Fat: 0g; Carbs: 31g; Protein: 1g; Calcium: 10mg; Sodium: 0mg; Potassium: 230mg; Phosphorus: 10mg

139. Grilled Pineapple with Cinnamon

Degree of difficulty: ★★☆☆☆

Preparation time: 10 mins

Cooking time: 5 mins

Servings: 2

Ingredients:

- 1 small pineapple, that is skinned, cored, and carved into rings
- 1/2 tsp ground cinnamon
- 1 tbsp honey

Directions:

1. Warm up your grill to med-high temp.
2. Brush the pineapple slices with a little honey on both sides.
3. Spray ground cinnamon on the pineapple slices.
4. Grill the pineapple for 2-3 mins on all sides, or 'til grill marks appear and the pineapple is mildly caramelized.
5. Take out from the grill then allow it to cool mildly.
6. Present the grilled pineapple with an extra spray of honey, if anticipated.

Per serving: Calories: 130kcal; Fat: 0g; Carbs: 34g; Protein: 1g; Calcium: 20mg; Sodium: 0mg; Potassium: 190mg; Phosphorus: 10mg

140. *Lemon Sorbet*

Degree of difficulty: ★★☆☆☆

Preparation time: 15 mins

Cooking time: 0 mins

Servings: 2

Ingredients:

- 1/2 teacup fresh lemon juice
- 1/4 teacup honey
- 1 teacup water
- Zest of one lemon (elective)

Directions:

1. Inside a container, blend the fresh lemon juice, honey, and water. Blend thoroughly till the sweetener is dissolved.
2. If anticipated, include the lemon zest for extra flavor.
3. Pour solution into an ice cream maker then churn using the manufacturer's instructions.
4. Once it reaches a sorbet consistency, transfer it to an airtight container and freeze for an extra 2 hrs to firm up.
5. Present the lemon sorbet.

Per serving: Calories: 150kcal; Fat: 0g; Carbs: 40g; Protein: 0g; Calcium: 10mg; Sodium: 5mg; Potassium: 80mg; Phosphorus: 10mg

141. *Rice Pudding*

Degree of difficulty: ★★☆☆☆

Preparation time: 5 mins

Cooking time: 25 mins

Servings: 2

Ingredients:

- 1/2 teacup cooked white rice
- 1 teacup low-fat milk
- 1/4 tsp ground cinnamon
- 1/4 tsp vanilla extract
- 1 tbsp honey

Directions:

1. Inside your saucepot, blend the cooked rice, milk, ground cinnamon, and vanilla extract.
2. Cook in a low heat, mixing regularly till the solution thickens, around 20-25 mins.
3. If you desire extra sweetness, stir in honey while the pudding is still warm.
4. Take out from temp. and allow it to cool.
5. Present chilled or at room temp.

Per serving: Calories: 180kcal; Fat: 2g; Carbs: 35g; Protein: 5g; Calcium: 180mg; Sodium: 80mg; Potassium: 250mg; Phosphorus: 150mg

142. *Carrot Cake Muffins*

Degree of difficulty: ★★☆☆☆

Preparation time: 15 mins

Cooking time: 25 mins

Servings: 2

Ingredients:

- 1 teacup grated carrots
- 1/2 teacup all-purpose flour
- 1/4 teacup almond flour
- 1/4 teacup low-sugar sweetener (e.g., erythritol or stevia)
- 1/2 tsp ground cinnamon
- 1/4 tsp ground nutmeg
- 1/2 tsp baking powder
- 1/4 tsp baking soda
- 1/4 teacup unsweetened applesauce
- 1/4 teacup low-fat milk
- 1 egg
- 1/2 tsp vanilla extract

Directions:

1. Warm up your oven to 350 deg.F.
2. Inside a container, blend grated carrots, all-purpose flour, almond flour, low-sugar sweetener, ground cinnamon, ground nutmeg, baking powder, and baking soda.
3. Inside an extra container, whisk collectively applesauce, milk, egg, and vanilla extract.
4. Mix wet and dry components 'til well blended.
5. Split the batter into muffin teacups.
6. Bake for 25 mins or 'til a toothpick comes out clean.
7. Allow the muffins to cool prior to presenting.

Per serving: Calories: 180kcal; Fat: 6g; Carbs: 28g; Protein: 5g; Calcium: 50mg; Sodium: 170mg; Potassium: 200mg; Phosphorus: 90mg

143. *Watermelon Popsicles*

Degree of difficulty: ★★☆☆☆

Preparation time: 10 mins

Cooking time: 0 mins

Servings: 2

Ingredients:

- 2 teacups fresh watermelon, seeds taken out and cubed
- 2 tbsps honey

Directions:

1. Place cubed watermelon and honey into a mixer.
2. Blend till you have a smooth liquid.
3. Pour watermelon solution into popsicle molds.
4. Insert popsicle sticks then freeze for 4 hrs or 'til completely frozen.
5. Run the molds briefly under warm water to release the popsicles.
6. Relish your refreshing watermelon popsicles.

Per serving: Calories: 80kcal; Fat: 0g; Carbs: 21g; Protein: 1g; Calcium: 10mg; Sodium: 0mg; Potassium: 200mg; Phosphorus: 10mg

144.   *Cinnamon and Walnut Oatmeal Bars*

Degree of difficulty: ★★☆☆☆
Preparation time: 15 mins
Cooking time: 30 mins
Servings: 2
Ingredients:

- 1 teacup rolled oats
- 1/4 teacup severed walnuts
- 1/4 teacup low-sugar sweetener (e.g., erythritol or stevia)
- 1/2 tsp ground cinnamon
- 1/4 tsp baking powder
- 1/4 teacup unsweetened applesauce
- 1/4 teacup low-fat milk
- 1 egg
- 1/2 tsp vanilla extract

Directions:

1. Warm up your oven to 350 deg.F.
2. Inside a container, blend rolled oats, severed walnuts, low-sugar sweetener, ground cinnamon, and baking powder.
3. Inside an extra container, whisk collectively applesauce, milk, egg, and vanilla extract.
4. Mix wet and dry components 'til well blended.
5. Transfer solution into an oiled baking dish.
6. Bake for 30 mins or 'til the bars are set and mildly browned.
7. Allow the oatmeal bars to cool and then cut them into squares.

Per serving: Calories: 220kcal; Fat: 9g; Carbs: 29g; Protein: 7g; Calcium: 70mg; Sodium: 150mg; Potassium: 240mg; Phosphorus: 100mg

145.   *Mango Slices with Lime*

Degree of difficulty: ★☆☆☆☆
Preparation time: 10 mins
Cooking time: 0 mins
Servings: 2
Ingredients:

- 1 ripe mango, skinned, eroded, and carved
- 1 lime, juiced

Directions:

1. Slice the ripe mango into thin, attractive slices.
2. Squeeze the juice of one lime over the mango slices.
3. Shake the mango carefully to cover it with lime juice.
4. Present your mango slices with a refreshing hint of lime.

Per serving: Calories: 80kcal; Fat: 0g; Carbs: 21g; Protein: 1g; Calcium: 10mg; Sodium: 0mg; Potassium: 190mg; Phosphorus: 10mg

146. *Strawberry Shortcake*

Degree of difficulty: ★★★☆☆

Preparation time: 15 mins

Cooking time: 20 mins

Servings: 2

Ingredients:

For the Shortcake:

- 1/2 teacup all-purpose flour
- 1/2 tsp baking powder
- 1 tbsp unsalted butter, softened
- 1/4 teacup low-fat milk
- 1/2 tsp vanilla extract
- 1 tbsp honey

For the Topping:

- 1 teacup fresh strawberries, carved
- 1/4 teacup low-fat whipped cream

Directions:

Shortcake:

1. Warm up your oven to 350 deg.F.
2. Inside a container, blend the flour and baking powder.
3. Inside a distinct container, mix the softened butter, milk, vanilla extract, and honey.
4. Blend wet and dry components then mix till a dough forms.
5. Split dough into two portions and shape them into biscuits.
6. Place biscuits on a baking sheet then bake for 15-20 mins or 'til they turn golden brown.

Topping:

7. While the shortcakes are baking, prepare the strawberries by slicing them.
8. Once the shortcakes have cooled, split them in half horizontally.
9. Place carved strawberries on the bottom half and include a dollop of low-fat whipped cream.
10. Place top half of the shortcake on the whipped cream to create a sandwich.
11. Present your low-sugar strawberry shortcake.

Per serving: Calories: 270kcal; Fat: 8g; Carbs: 46g; Protein: 5g; Calcium: 100mg; Sodium: 20mg; Potassium: 270mg; Phosphorus: 120mg

147. *Carrot and Pineapple Cake*

Degree of difficulty: ★★★☆☆

Preparation time: 20 mins

Cooking time: 35 mins

Servings: 2

Ingredients:

- 1 teacup grated carrots
- 1/2 teacup crushed pineapple (tinned, in juice, drained)
- 1/4 teacup unsweetened applesauce
- 1/4 teacup brown sugar
- 1/4 teacup vegetable oil
- 1/2 teacup all-purpose flour
- 1/4 teacup wheat flour
- 1/2 tsp baking soda
- 1/2 tsp ground cinnamon
- 1/4 tsp ground nutmeg
- Cooking spray

Directions:

1. Warm up oven to 350 deg.F then oil a small baking dish.
2. Inside a container, blend grated carrots, crushed pineapple, unsweetened applesauce, brown sugar, and vegetable oil. Blend thoroughly.
3. Inside an extra container, whisk collectively all-purpose flour, wheat flour, baking soda, ground cinnamon, and ground nutmeg.
4. Gradually include the dry components to the carrot solution then stir till just blended.
5. Pour batter into your prepared baking dish.
6. Bake into your warmed up oven for 30-35 mins or 'til a toothpick placed into the center comes out clean.
7. Allow the Carrot and Pineapple Cake to cool prior to presenting.

Per serving: Calories: 400kcal; Fat: 20g; Carbs: 50g; Protein: 5g; Calcium: 40mg; Sodium: 170mg; Potassium: 300mg; Phosphorus: 100mg

148. *Baked Pears with Cinnamon*

Degree of difficulty: ★★☆☆☆

Preparation time: 10 mins

Cooking time: 20 mins

Servings: 2

Ingredients:

- 2 ripe pears, divided and cored
- 1 tbsp lemon juice
- 1/2 tsp ground cinnamon
- 1/4 teacup honey
- Cooking spray

Directions:

1. Warm up oven to 375 deg.F then oil a baking dish.
2. Brush the pear halves using lemon juice and put them in the baking dish.
3. Spray ground cinnamon over the pears.
4. Spray honey over the pears.
5. Bake into your warmed up oven for 20 mins or 'til the pears are soft and caramelized.
6. Present the Baked Pears with Cinnamon warm.

Per serving: Calories: 180kcal; Fat: 0g; Carbs: 48g; Protein: 1g; Calcium: 10mg; Sodium: 0mg; Potassium: 210mg; Phosphorus: 20mg

149.   *Lemon and Honey Panna Cotta*

Degree of difficulty: ★★★☆☆

Preparation time: 15 mins

Cooking time: 10 mins

Chilling Time: 2-3 hrs

Servings: 2

Ingredients:

- 1 teacup low-fat milk
- 1 tsp unflavored gelatin
- 2 tbsps honey
- Zest and juice of 1 lemon
- 1/2 teacup plain Greek yogurt

Directions:

1. Inside a mini container, spray gelatin over 1/4 teacup of cold milk. Allow it to relax for a couple of mins to bloom.
2. Inside your saucepot, heat the remaining 3/4 teacup of milk at low temp. till it's warm but not boiling.
3. Stir in honey and lemon zest till dissolved.
4. Put the bloomed gelatin to the warm milk solution then stir till fully dissolved.
5. Take out from temp. then stir in your lemon juice.
6. Let the solution to cool mildly, then whisk in plain Greek yogurt.
7. Transfer the solution into serving glasses or ramekins.
8. Chill in the fridge for 2-3 hrs or 'til set.
9. Present the Lemon and Honey Panna Cotta chilled.

Per serving: Calories: 200kcal; Fat: 2g; Carbs: 34g; Protein: 11g; Calcium: 180mg; Sodium: 60mg; Potassium: 220mg; Phosphorus: 180mg

150.   *Peach Cobbler*

Degree of difficulty: ★★☆☆☆

Preparation time: 15 mins

Cooking time: 30 mins

Servings: 2

Ingredients:

- 2 teacups tinned peaches (in juice, drained)
- 1/2 teacup all-purpose flour
- 1/4 teacup wheat flour
- 1/4 teacup sugar (or a renal-friendly sweetener)
- 1/2 tsp baking powder
- 1/4 tsp salt
- 1/2 teacup low-fat milk
- 1/4 tsp vanilla extract
- Cooking spray

Directions:

1. Warm up oven to 375 deg.F and oil a baking dish.
2. Organize the drained tinned peaches in the baking dish.
3. Inside a container, whisk collectively all-purpose flour, wheat flour, sugar, baking powder, and salt.
4. Stir in low-fat milk and vanilla extract till a batter forms.
5. Pour batter over the peaches in the baking dish.
6. Bake in to your warmed up oven for 30 mins or 'til the cobbler is golden and the peach filling is bubbly.
7. Present the Peach Cobbler warm.

Per serving: Calories: 320kcal; Fat: 1g; Carbs: 75g; Protein: 6g; Calcium: 60mg; Sodium: 330mg; Potassium: 460mg; Phosphorus: 80mg

CHAPTER 5: WEEKLY Shopping List

Compiling a weekly shopping list is a vital component of sustaining a nutritious and well-balanced diet, particularly for individuals with specific dietary needs, such as those following a renal diet. When planning your weekly shopping list, it's crucial to select foods that align with your dietary restrictions and can be used efficiently throughout the week to minimize waste. In the case of a renal diet, this means focusing on fresh vegetables and fruits that are low in sodium, potassium, and phosphorus. Additionally, the shopping list should be suitable for a 30-day meal plan, ensuring that you have all the necessary components for a month's worth of renal-friendly meals.

Individuals with kidney disease or impaired kidney function need to pay close attention to their diet to manage their condition effectively. A renal-friendly shopping list ensures that you have the right foods on hand to support your kidney health. The goal is to reduce the intake of substances like sodium, potassium, and phosphorus, which can be harmful to the kidneys when consumed in extra. By selecting the appropriate foods during your weekly shopping trips, you can better control your nutrient intake and minimize the risk of complications associated with kidney disease.

What to Eat and What to Avoid

What to Include in Your Renal-Friendly Weekly Shopping List

Fresh Vegetables

- Cabbage
- Cauliflower
- Celery
- Broccoli
- Brussels Sprouts
- Red bell peppers
- Zucchini
- Green beans
- Eggplant
- Onions (in moderation)
- Radishes
- Lettuce (romaine or iceberg)
- Kale
- Spinach (in moderation)
- Cucumbers
- Artichoke
- Asparagus

Fresh Fruits

- Apples (skinned and carved)
- Cranberries
- Blueberries
- Raspberries
- Pineapple
- Red or black grapes
- Watermelon
- Mango
- Cherries (in moderation)
- Peaches (in moderation)
- Pears (in moderation)
- Plums (in moderation)

Legumes

- Beans (such as black beans, kidney beans)
- Chickpeas
- Lentils
- Peas

Lean Proteins

- Skinless chicken breast
- Turkey (skinless)
- White fish (cod, haddock, or flounder)
- Eggs (egg whites recommended)
- Lean cuts of beef (in moderation)

Grains and Starches

- White rice
- White bread
- Pasta (in moderation)
- Rice cakes (plain or low-sodium varieties)
- Cereal (low-potassium, low-phosphorus)
- Flour (for baking)

Dairy and Dairy Alternatives

- Low-fat or fat-free milk
- Low-fat or fat-free yogurt
- Dairy-free milk alternatives (e.g., almond milk or rice milk)
- Dairy-free yogurt alternatives (low-potassium varieties)

Condiments and Seasonings

- Fresh or dried herbs and spices (e.g., basil, oregano, thyme, rosemary)

- Vinegar (apple cider, balsamic, or white)
- Lemon juice (in moderation)
- Low-sodium soy sauce or tamari
- Low-sodium broth or bouillon

Snacks and Sweets

- Rice cakes
- Sorbet (in moderation)
- Homemade baked goods (using renal-friendly components)

Beverages

- Water
- Herbal teas (avoid high-potassium varieties)
- Coffee (in moderation)
- Carbonated water (plain or low-sodium)

What to Avoid on Your Renal-Friendly Shopping List

In addition to knowing what to include, it's equally important to be aware of foods and components to avoid when following a renal diet. Here's what to skip:

High-Sodium Foods

- Processed and tinned foods (e.g., tinned soups, tinned vegetables)
- Pre-packaged snacks (chips, pretzels)
- Processed meats (bacon, sausages, deli meats)
- High-sodium condiments (soy sauce, teriyaki sauce)
- Fast food and restaurant meals

High-Potassium Foods

- Bananas
- Oranges and orange juice
- Potatoes
- Tomatoes and tomato products (sauce, paste)
- Dried fruits (raisins, prunes)
- Avocado
- Melons (cantaloupe, honeydew)
- Spinach and other high-potassium vegetables

High-Phosphorus Foods

- Dairy products (milk, cheese, yogurt)
- Nuts and seeds
- Colas and dark sodas
- Chocolate
- Processed and convenience foods

- Whole grains (brown rice, whole wheat bread)

High-Protein Foods (in excess)

- Red meat
- Poultry with skin
- Fish (especially high-purine varieties)
- Eggs (limit yolks)
- Organ meats (liver, kidney)

Excessive Fluids

- While water is essential, excessive fluid intake can be harmful. Follow your healthcare provider's recommendations for daily fluid limits.
- **Alcohol**: Alcohol can be taxing on the kidneys, so it's best to limit or avoid it.

Additional Tips for Efficient Weekly Shopping

1. **Buy Frozen and Canned Options:** While fresh fruits and vegetables are ideal, it's also practical to have some frozen or low-sodium tinned options on hand for times when you need a quick meal or don't have access to fresh produce.
2. **Consider Batch Cooking:** Preparing larger quantities of renal-friendly dishes and freezing them in portions can save time and reduce waste. It ensures that you always have a ready-made meal available.
3. **Be Mindful of Leftovers:** Plan meals that allow you to repurpose leftovers creatively. For example, roast chicken can become chicken salad or chicken stir-fry in later meals.
4. **Check for Sales & Discounts:** Look for sales and discounts on renal-friendly items and non-perishables, and consider buying in bulk when possible.
5. **Create a Shopping Routine:** Establish a regular shopping routine, whether it's weekly, bi-weekly, or monthly, to ensure you always have fresh components on hand for your renal-friendly meals.

Incorporating Variety into Your Renal Diet

Maintaining a renal-friendly diet doesn't mean sacrificing variety or flavor in your meals. You can explore different recipes and cooking techniques to keep your meals exciting and enjoyable. Here are some ideas:

1. **Explore Different Cooking Methods:** Try grilling, roasting, steaming, or sautéing your vegetables to bring out unique flavors and textures.
2. **Experiment with Herbs and Spices:** A diverse array of herbs and spices can introduce depth and richness to your culinary creations without relying on excessive salt or sodium.
3. **Get Creative with Seasonings:** Use low-sodium seasonings and condiments like vinegar, lemon juice, and low-sodium soy sauce to create flavorful marinades and dressings.
4. **Try New Grains:** While white rice is a staple in a renal diet, you can experiment with other low-potassium grains like couscous, bulgur, or quinoa.
5. **Discover Dairy Alternatives:** Explore dairy-free milk and yogurt alternatives to find the ones that suit your taste and dietary restrictions.

6. **Relish Limited Portions of High-Potassium Foods:** While some high-potassium foods should be avoided or limited, you can still relish them in controlled portions. For example, a small serving of berries can be a delightful treat.

CHAPTER 6: 30 Day Meal Plan

Designing a 30-day meal plan tailored for individuals following a renal diet requires careful consideration of nutritional needs, restrictions, and health goals. This specialized diet is essential for individuals with kidney-related issues, and it aims to manage and reduce the burden on the kidneys. Adhering to a renal diet can significantly impact a person's overall health, especially in the case of men and women, who may have differing nutritional requirements and preferences. Therefore, creating distinct meal plans for men and women can help cater to their specific dietary needs while ensuring optimal health and well-being.

Meal Plan Tailored for Men

When creating a meal plan tailored for men, it's essential to consider their unique nutritional needs, which often differ from those of women. Men typically have higher caloric requirements due to their larger body size and muscle mass. They also have different nutritional needs for certain vitamins and minerals. However, the emphasis should still be on controlling sodium, potassium, and phosphorus intake. Here's a sample 30-day meal plan for men that focuses on meeting these needs while promoting overall health and well-being.

Day	Breakfast	Snack	Lunch and Appetizers	Snack	Dinner and Appetizers
1	Chia Pudding with Berries	Cheese and Whole Wheat Crackers	Turkey and Cranberry Sandwich, Lentil Soup	Sliced Cucumber with Lemon	Teriyaki Tofu with Steamed Broccoli, Guacamole with Veggie Sticks
2	Blueberry Muffins	Popcorn	Chicken and Wild Rice Soup, Deviled Eggs	Fresh Fruit Salad	Grilled Swordfish with Lemon Butter, Caprese Skewers
3	Oatmeal with Berries	Watermelon Cubes	Zucchini Noodles with Pesto, Caprese Quinoa Salad	Carrot Sticks with Hummus	Lemon Herb Tilapia, Roasted Brussels Sprouts
4	Waffle with Peach Compote	Fig and Walnut Bites	Quinoa Stuffed Peppers, Roasted Garlic Cauliflower	Cottage Cheese and Sliced Peaches	Baked Eggplant Parmesan, Mixed Greens with Raspberry Vinaigrette
5	Quinoa Breakfast Bowl	Berries with Whipped Cream	Egg Salad Lettuce Wraps, Greek Potato Salad	Pita Bread with Hummus	Baked Lemon Chicken, Green Bean Almondine
6	Zucchini and Carrot Pancakes	Sliced Bell Peppers	Baked Salmon with Lemon-Dill Sauce, Rice Pilaf	Dried Apricots	Vegetable and Bean Chili , Steamed

Day	Breakfast	Snack	Lunch and Appetizers	Snack	Dinner and Appetizers
			with Mixed Veggies		Asparagus with Lemon
7	Mango Smoothie	Carrot Sticks with Hummus	Turkey and Vegetable Stir-Fry, Mashed Cauliflower	Watermelon Cubes	Seared Tofu with Ginger Glaze, Roasted Brussels Sprouts
8	Homemade Wheat Bran Cereal	Fig and Ricotta Bruschetta	Grilled Chicken Salad, Lemon-Dill Cucumber Salad	Baked Apple Chip	Quinoa and Chickpea Pilaf, Caprese Skewers
9	Pears with Ricotta Cheese	Pomegranate Granita	Sea Bass with Cilantro Pesto, Spinach and Feta Stuffed Mushrooms	Celery and Peanut Butter	Grilled Pork Tenderloin, Baked Artichoke Hearts
10	Breakfast Couscous	Berries with Whipped Cream	Quinoa and Black Bean Salad, Baked Zucchini Chips	Carrot Cake Muffins	Grilled Swordfish with Lemon Butter, Roasted Garlic Cauliflower
11	Blueberry and Lemon Yogurt Parfait	Pita Bread with Hummus	Tuna Salad Wraps, Greek Potato Salad	Fresh Fruit Salad	Turkey and Mushroom Risotto, Roasted Brussels Sprouts
12	Quinoa and Apple Porridge	Carrot and Celery Sticks with Hummus	Quinoa Stuffed Peppers, Guacamole with Veggie Sticks	Hard-Boiled Eggs	Baked Cod with Herbs, Deviled Roasted Beet Salad
13	Veggie Omelet	Cheese and Whole Wheat Crackers	Lentil Soup, Roasted Eggplant Dip	Berries with Whipped Cream	Lemon Herb Tilapia, Baked Artichoke Hearts
14	Pineapple and Coconut Milk Rice	Sliced Cucumber with Lemon	Turkey and Cranberry Sandwich, Caprese Quinoa Salad	Popcorn	Seared Tofu with Ginger Glaze, Caprese Skewers
15	Greek Yogurt with Mixed Berries	Watermelon Cubes	Baked Salmon with Lemon-Dill Sauce, Spinach and Feta Stuffed Mushrooms	Dried Apricots	Balsamic Glazed Salmon, Roasted Garlic Cauliflower
16	Apple Cinnamon Pancakes	Fresh Fruit Salad	Grilled Shrimp and Asparagus,	Celery and Peanut Butter	Teriyaki Tofu with Steamed Broccoli, Deviled Eggs

Day	Breakfast	Snack	Lunch and Appetizers	Snack	Dinner and Appetizers
			Lemon-Dill Cucumber Salad		
17	Carrot and Pineapple Cake	Fig and Walnut Bites	Tofu and Vegetable Stir-Fry, Roasted Eggplant Dip	Dried Apricots	Seared Tofu with Ginger Glaze, Caprese Skewers
18	Chia Pudding with Berries	Berries with Whipped Cream	Caprese Salad with Balsamic Glaze, Deviled Eggs	Pita Bread with Hummus	Baked Chicken Breast with Herbs, Roasted Brussels Sprouts
19	Oatmeal with Berries	Baked Zucchini Chips	Quinoa Stuffed Peppers, Rice Pilaf with Mixed Veggies	Cheese and Whole Wheat Crackers	Grilled Swordfish with Lemon Butter, Caprese Skewers
20	Berry and Banana Smoothie Bowl	Pita Bread with Hummus	Egg Salad Lettuce Wraps, Guacamole with Veggie Sticks	Fresh Fruit Salad	Quinoa and Chickpea Pilaf, Spinach and Feta Stuffed Mushrooms
21	Waffle with Peach Compote	Popcorn	Turkey and Vegetable Stir-Fry, Roasted Garlic Cauliflower	Sliced Cucumber with Lemon	Baked Lemon Chicken, Deviled Eggs
22	Pears with Ricotta Cheese	Watermelon Cubes	Sea Bass with Cilantro Pesto, Caprese Quinoa Salad	Carrot Sticks with Hummus	Teriyaki Tofu with Steamed Broccoli, Baked Artichoke Hearts
23	Breakfast Couscous	Greek Yogurt with Honey	Chicken and Wild Rice Soup, Spinach and Feta Stuffed Mushrooms	Berries with Whipped Cream	Beef and Barley Soup Roasted Brussels Sprouts
24	Blueberry and Lemon Yogurt Parfait	Dried Apricots	Tuna Salad Wraps, Lemon-Dill Cucumber Salad	Baked Zucchini Chips	Baked Cod with Herbs, Caprese Skewers
25	Quinoa and Apple Porridge	Berries with Whipped Cream	Lentil Soup, Roasted Eggplant Dip	Pita Bread with Hummus	Seared Tofu with Ginger Glaze, Deviled Eggs
26	Veggie Omelet	Fresh Fruit Salad	Turkey and Cranberry Sandwich,	Edamame	Teriyaki Tofu with Steamed Broccoli,

Day	Breakfast	Snack	Lunch and Appetizers	Snack	Dinner and Appetizers
			Caprese Quinoa Salad		Guacamole with Veggie Sticks
27	Pineapple and Coconut Milk Rice	Sliced Cucumber with Lemon	Baked Salmon with Lemon-Dill Sauce, Rice Pilaf with Mixed Veggies	Cottage Cheese and Sliced Peaches	Grilled Swordfish with Lemon Butter, Roasted Garlic Cauliflower
28	Greek Yogurt with Mixed Berries	Watermelon Cubes	Grilled Shrimp and Asparagus, Spinach and Feta Stuffed Mushrooms	Dried Apricots	Balsamic Glazed Salmon, Caprese Skewers
29	Apple Cinnamon Pancakes	Pita Bread with Hummus	Caprese Salad with Balsamic Glaze, Deviled Eggs	Cheese and Whole Wheat Crackers	Baked Chicken Breast with Herbs, Roasted Brussels Sprouts
30	Zucchini and Carrot Pancakes	Fig and Walnut Bites	Quinoa Stuffed Peppers, Roasted Garlic Cauliflower	Fresh Fruit Salad	Grilled Swordfish with Lemon Butter, Guacamole with Veggie Sticks

Meal Plan Tailored for Women

Women have unique nutritional requirements that can change during different life stages, such as pregnancy, lactation, and menopause. This meal plan will focus on the general nutritional needs of women, promoting overall health and well-being.

Day	Breakfast	Snack	Lunch and Appetizers	Snack	Dinner and Appetizers
1	Chia Pudding with Berries	Celery and Peanut Butter	Turkey and Cranberry Sandwich, Caprese Quinoa Salad	Carrot Sticks with Hummus	Teriyaki Tofu with Steamed Broccoli, Guacamole with Veggie Sticks
2	Blueberry Muffins	Fresh Fruit Salad	Lentil Soup, Roasted Eggplant Dip	Berries with Whipped Cream	Grilled Swordfish with Lemon Butter, Caprese Skewers
3	Oatmeal with Berries	Sliced Cucumber with Lemon	Turkey and Cranberry Sandwich, Caprese Salad	Pita Bread with Hummus	Baked Lemon Chicken, Roasted Brussels Sprouts

Day	Breakfast	Snack	Lunch and Appetizers	Snack	Dinner and Appetizers
4	Waffle with Peach Compote	Cheese and Whole Wheat Crackers	Quinoa Stuffed Peppers, Roasted Garlic Cauliflower	Mango Slices with Lime	Beef and Barley Soup, Steamed Asparagus with Lemon
5	Berry and Banana Smoothie Bowl	Watermelon Cubes	Egg Salad Lettuce Wraps, Greek Potato Salad	Sliced Bell Peppers	Chickpea Salad, Baked Artichoke Hearts
6	Zucchini and Carrot Pancakes	Fig and Walnut Bites	Baked Salmon with Lemon-Dill Sauce, Spinach and Feta Stuffed Mushrooms	Dried Apricots	Teriyaki Tofu with Steamed Broccoli, Caprese Skewers
7	Mango Smoothie	Carrot Sticks with Hummus	Turkey and Vegetable Stir-Fry, Mashed Cauliflower	Watermelon Cubes	Vegetable and Bean Chili, Roasted Brussels Sprouts
8	Homemade Wheat Bran Cereal	Fig and Ricotta Bruschetta	Grilled Chicken Salad, Lemon-Dill Cucumber Salad	Sliced Cucumber with Lemon	Quinoa and Chickpea Pilaf, Deviled Eggs
9	Pears with Ricotta Cheese	Pomegranate Granita	Sea Bass with Cilantro Pesto, Caprese Quinoa Salad	Grilled Pineapple with Cinnamon	Grilled Pork Tenderloin, Baked Artichoke Hearts
10	Breakfast Couscous	Berries with Whipped Cream	Chicken and Wild Rice Soup, Baked Zucchini Chips	Watermelon Popsicles	Baked Lemon Chicken, Roasted Garlic Cauliflower
11	Blueberry and Lemon Yogurt Parfait	Pita Bread with Hummus	Tuna Salad Wraps, Lemon-Dill Cucumber Salad	Fresh Fruit Salad	Teriyaki Tofu with Steamed Broccoli, Deviled Eggs
12	Quinoa and Apple Porridge	Carrot and Celery Sticks with Hummus	Chicken and Wild Rice Soup, Pear and Walnut Salad	Sliced Cucumber with Lemon	Baked Cod with Herbs, Caprese Skewers
13	Veggie Omelet	Berries with Whipped Cream	Lentil Soup, Roasted Eggplant Dip	Edamame	Lemon Herb Tilapia, Caprese Skewers
14	Pineapple and Coconut Milk Rice	Sliced Cucumber with Lemon	Turkey and Cranberry Sandwich, Caprese Salad	Popcorn	Mango and Black Bean Salad, Baked Artichoke Hearts

Day	Breakfast	Snack	Lunch and Appetizers	Snack	Dinner and Appetizers
15	Greek Yogurt with Mixed Berries	Watermelon Cubes	Baked Salmon with Lemon-Dill Sauce, Spinach and Feta Stuffed Mushrooms	Dried Apricots	Balsamic Glazed Salmon, Roasted Garlic Cauliflower
16	Apple Cinnamon Pancakes	Fresh Fruit Salad	Grilled Shrimp and Asparagus, Lemon-Dill Cucumber Salad	Carrot Sticks with Hummus	Grilled Swordfish with Lemon Butter, Caesar Salad with Croutons
17	Zucchini and Carrot Pancakes	Fig and Walnut Bites	Minestrone Soup, Deviled Eggs	Dried Apricots	Seared Tofu with Ginger Glaze, Caprese Skewers
18	Chia Pudding with Berries	Berries with Whipped Cream	Chickpea and Cucumber Wrap, Caprese Salad with Balsamic Glaze	Pita Bread with Hummus	Baked Chicken Breast with Herbs, Roasted Brussels Sprouts
19	Oatmeal with Berries	Hard-Boiled Eggs	Quinoa Stuffed Peppers, Rice Pilaf with Mixed Veggies	Cheese and Whole Wheat Crackers	Lemon Herb Tilapia, Caprese Skewers
20	Berry and Banana Smoothie Bowl	Pita Bread with Hummus	Egg Salad Lettuce Wraps, Asian Cabbage Salad	Fresh Fruit Salad	Quinoa and Chickpea Pilaf, Spinach and Feta Stuffed Mushrooms
21	Waffle with Peach Compote	Popcorn	Turkey and Vegetable Stir-Fry, Roasted Garlic Cauliflower	Sliced Cucumber with Lemon	Baked Lemon Chicken, Caesar Salad with Croutons
22	Carrot Cake Muffins	Watermelon Cubes	Sea Bass with Cilantro Pesto, Caprese Quinoa Salad	Carrot Sticks with Hummus	Teriyaki Tofu with Steamed Broccoli, Baked Artichoke Hearts
23	Breakfast Couscous	Cheese and Whole Wheat Crackers	White Fish soup, Spinach and Feta Stuffed Mushrooms	Berries with Whipped Cream	Chicken and Wild Rice Soup, Roasted Brussels Sprouts
24	Blueberry and Lemon Yogurt Parfait	Dried Apricots	Tuna Salad Wraps, Lemon-	Hard-Boiled Eggs	Baked Cod with Herbs, Caprese Skewers

Day	Breakfast	Snack	Lunch and Appetizers	Snack	Dinner and Appetizers
			Dill Cucumber Salad		
25	Quinoa and Apple Porridge	Berries with Whipped Cream	Lentil Soup, Roasted Eggplant Dip	Pita Bread with Hummus	Seared Tofu with Ginger Glaze, Apple and Cranberry Coleslaw
26	Veggie Omelet	Fresh Fruit Salad	Turkey and Cranberry Sandwich, Caprese Quinoa Salad	Sliced Cucumber with Lemon	Lemon Dill Chicken, Guacamole with Veggie Sticks
27	Pineapple and Coconut Milk Rice	Sliced Cucumber with Lemon	Baked Salmon with Lemon-Dill Sauce, Rice Pilaf with Mixed Veggies	Cottage Cheese and Sliced Peaches	Grilled Swordfish with Lemon Butter, Roasted Garlic Cauliflower
28	Greek Yogurt with Mixed Berries	Watermelon Cubes	Grilled Shrimp and Asparagus, Spinach and Feta Stuffed Mushrooms	Dried Apricots	Balsamic Glazed Salmon, Caprese Skewers
29	Apple Cinnamon Pancakes	Pita Bread with Hummus	Caprese Salad with Balsamic Glaze; Deviled Eggs	Cheese and Whole Wheat Crackers	Baked Chicken Breast with Herbs, Roasted Brussels Sprouts
30	Zucchini and Carrot Pancakes	Fig and Walnut Bites	Quinoa Stuffed Peppers, Roasted Garlic Cauliflower	Fresh Fruit Salad	Lemon Herb Tilapia, Guacamole with Veggie Sticks

Conversion Chart

Volume Equivalents (Liquid)

US Standard	US Standard (oz.)	Metric (approximate)
2 tbsps	1 fl. oz.	30 milliliter
¼ teacup	2 fl. oz.	60 milliliter
½ teacup	4 fl. oz.	120 milliliter
1 teacup	8 fl. oz.	240 milliliter
1½ teacups	12 fl. oz.	355 milliliter
2 teacups or 1 pint	16 fl. oz.	475 milliliter
4 teacups or 1 quart	32 fl. oz.	1 Liter
1 gallon	128 fl. oz.	4 Liter

Volume Equivalents (Dry)

US Standard	Metric (approximate)
⅛ tsp	0.5 milliliter
¼ tsp	1 milliliter
½ tsp	2 milliliter
¾ tsp	4 milliliter
1 tsp	5 milliliter
1 tbsp	15 milliliter
¼ teacup	59 milliliter
⅓ teacup	79 milliliter
½ teacup	118 milliliter
⅔ teacup	156 milliliter
¾ teacup	177 milliliter
1 teacup	235 milliliter
2 teacups or 1 pint	475 milliliter
3 teacups	700 milliliter
4 teacups or 1 quart	1 Liter

Oven Temperatures

Fahrenheit (F)	Celsius (C) (approximate)
250 deg.F	120 deg.C
300 deg.F	150 deg.C
325 deg.F	165 deg.C
350 deg.F	180 deg.C
375 deg.F	190 deg.C

400 deg.F	200 deg.C
425 deg.F	220 deg.C
450 deg.F	230 deg.C

Weight Equivalents

US Standard	Metric (approximate)
1 tbsp	15 g
½ oz.	15 g
1 oz.	30 g
2 oz.	60 g
4 oz.	115 g
8 oz.	225 g
12 oz.	340 g
16 oz. or 1 lb.	455 g

Conclusion

The renal diet is a specialized nutritional plan designed for individuals with compromised kidney function, typically those suffering from chronic kidney disease (CKD) or other renal conditions. Its primary goal is to help manage the progression of kidney disease and alleviate associated symptoms by regulating the intake of certain nutrients and fluids. A well-managed renal diet can help control electrolyte imbalances, reduce the workload on the kidneys, and minimize the accumulation of waste products in the blood. Key components often include controlling the intake of sodium, potassium, phosphorus, and protein, while ensuring adequate calorie intake to prevent malnutrition. Implementing the renal diet, along with other recommended medical treatments, can significantly improve the quality of life and overall health outcomes for individuals with renal issues. However, it is crucial for patients to work closely with healthcare professionals, including registered dietitians, to create a personalized plan that considers their specific nutritional needs and medical requirements.

I highly recommend exploring the recipes within this book, as they offer a diverse array of delicious and kidney-friendly meals that can be simply incorporated into your daily routine. These recipes have been thoughtfully crafted to not only adhere to the requirements of a renal diet but also to tantalize your taste buds and provide you with a culinary journey that supports your health goals. Embrace these flavorful dishes as a step toward a more vibrant, fulfilling, and kidney-friendly lifestyle.

Index

Lentil Soup, 36
Mackerel and Potato Salad, 71
Mango and Black Bean Salad, 72
Mango Slices with Lime, 99
Mango Smoothie, 22
Mashed Cauliflower, 88
Minestrone Soup, 41
Mixed Berry Compote, 94
Mixed Green Salad with Lemon Vinaigrette, 61
Mixed Greens with Raspberry Vinaigrette, 64
Mushroom and Pea Risotto, 44
Oatmeal with Berries, 23
Peach Cobbler, 102
Peach Sorbet, 95
Pear and Walnut Salad, 63
Pears with Ricotta Cheese, 24
Pineapple and Coconut Milk Rice, 31
Pita Bread with Hummus, 78
Poached Pears in Red Wine, 91
Pomegranate Granita, 93
Popcorn, 79
Pumpkin Custard, 93
Quinoa and Apple Porridge, 29
Quinoa and Black Bean Salad, 65
Quinoa and Chickpea Pilaf, 53
Quinoa and Roasted Vegetable Salad, 72
Quinoa Breakfast Bowl, 21
Quinoa Stuffed Peppers, 37
Ratatouille with Rice, 50
Rice Cakes with Almond Butter, 80
Rice Pilaf with Mixed Veggies, 84
Rice Pudding, 97
Roasted Beet Salad, 63

Roasted Brussels Sprouts, 89
Roasted Eggplant Dip, 83
Roasted Garlic Cauliflower, 90
Roasted Red Pepper Salad, 67
Roasted Vegetable Wrap, 40
Sea Bass with Cilantro Pesto, 38
Seared Tofu with Ginger Glaze, 46
Shrimp and Vegetable Kebabs, 53
Sliced Bell Peppers, 81
Sliced Cucumber with Lemon, 76
Spaghetti Squash with Marinara, 57
Spinach and Feta Stuffed Mushrooms, 86
Spinach and Strawberry Salad, 65
Steamed Asparagus with Lemon, 90
Strawberry Shortcake, 99
Teriyaki Tofu with Steamed Broccoli, 49
Tofu and Edamame Salad, 68
Tofu and Vegetable Stir-Fry, 39
Tuna Salad Wraps, 34
Turkey and Cranberry Sandwich, 32
Turkey and Mushroom Risotto, 49
Turkey and Rice Casserole, 55
Turkey and Vegetable Stir-Fry, 34
Vegetable and Bean Chili, 61
Vegetable Curry with Basmati Rice, 58
Veggie Omelet, 22
Waffle with Peach Compote, 25
Watermelon and Feta Salad, 70
Watermelon Cubes, 76
Watermelon Popsicles, 98
White Fish soup, 42
Zucchini and Carrot Pancakes, 28
Zucchini Noodles with Pesto, 33

Copyright - Elisa Cooper – All rights reserved.

www.ingramcontent.com/pod-product-compliance
Lightning Source LLC
Chambersburg PA
CBHW081604270726
48661CB00020B/3687